HANDY CHARTING GUIDELINES FOR NURSING FACILITIES

Written and edited by
Ann G Uniack, RHIA

From CMS State Operations Manual
Pub 100-07 Appendix PP
Guidance to Surveyors for
Long Term Care Facilities
and
Code of Federal Regulations
Section 483.25 Quality of Care

S.N.A.P., Inc
Skilled Nursing Assessment Programs
P.O. Box 574
San Anselmo, CA 94979
(415) 453-6029

First Printing, March 2006

Printed in the United States of America

Published by: SNAP, Inc., P.O. Box 574, San Anselmo, CA 94979. Additional copies of this book may be ordered from the publisher. Prepaid orders only. Checks made payable to SNAP in the amount of $29.95. Add $4.00 to cover handling and postage. California residents include 7.75% ($2.32) sales tax.

ISBN # 1-881671-28-3 and 978-1-881671-28-2

Index

INTRODUCTION

Time and again we hear the old adage: "If it wasn't charted, it wasn't done". However, knowing what to say and when to say it, may truly be the secret.

Resident care involves a team of health care professionals. All rely on the clinical record for complete, reliable information to make decisions. To be useful the clinical record must be organized in a concise, consistent and retrievable manner. Accurate and timely documentation results in quality care. Lack of documentation can result in poor care.

Handy Charting Guidelines for Nursing Facilities provides a framework for documenting resident care. These guidelines enable all staff disciplines to assess the resident's problems and needs and clearly document that quality care has been given to each resident.

1. Federal Regulations

The federal regulations for nursing facilities, commonly known as OBRA, are written to improve quality of care in nursing facilities. Not only do the regulations address resident rights and specify a comprehensive resident assessment system; but also, these regulations require that care and services be provided so that each resident may attain their ***"highest practicable well-being".***

The chapters in this book are organized to identify:

- Federal regulations,
- Quality measures and indicators calculated from Minimum Data Set (MDS) data,
- Definitions,
- Surveyor clinical guidance,
- Procedures that surveyors use to evaluate care, and
- A specific charting outline for:
  interdisciplinary team (IDT) input,
  assessment,
  orders,
  care plan and
  narrative notes.

2. Quality Measures/Indicators

Quality measures and indicators give information about the care in a nursing facility, such as the number of falls, pressure ulcers, and how many residents have lost too much weight. They are calculated from data submitted to State survey agencies. The facility has access to these calculations through their State MDS Transmission Website.

Quality measures are a subset of these calculations and are reported on the Center for Medicare and Medicaid Services (CMS) website "Nursing Home Compare." The quality measures are available to the public to assist them in making a decision about a facility when choosing a nursing home for themselves or for others.

During the preparation tasks prior to survey, the quality

indicators are used to identify facility problems and/or focus areas. The facility is wise to review these data on an on-going basis, and make sure that the information reported is accurate. Quality measures and indicators should be evaluated as part of the facility quality assessment and assurance program to identify trends and opportunities for quality improvement.

3. Definitions

CMS provides definitions and clarification of term used in the surveyor guidance. For example, Federal Regulations state that the intent of Section 483.25 Quality of Care is that:

- each resident is to attain the "**highest practicable**" physical, mental, and psychosocial well-being.
- the resident's condition will not deteriorate unless **"unavoidable diminution"** is documented in the clinical record.

The following definitions are provided by CMS:

Highest practicable

The highest level of functioning and well-being possible, limited only by the individual's presenting functional status and potential for improvement or reduced rate of functional decline. Highest practicable is determined through the comprehensive resident assessment by competently and thoroughly addressing the physical, mental or psychosocial needs of the individual.

Unavoidable diminution

*Conditions demonstrating **"unavoidable diminution"** in resident condition include:*

1. The natural progression of the resident's disease;

2. *Deterioration of the resident's physical condition associated with the onset of a physical or mental disability while receiving care to restore or maintain functional abilities;*

3. *The resident's or his/her surrogate's or representative's refusal of care and treatment to restore or maintain functional abilities after aggressive efforts by the facility to counsel and/or offer alternatives to the resident, surrogate, or representative. Refusal of such care and treatment should be documented in the clinical record.*

4. Surveyor Guidance

CMS provides clinical guidance to surveyors to evaluate the quality of care provided to residents. In each chapter, this book presents the key points in the clinical guidance to provide a reference for documentation.

The clinical guidance is based on the Resident Assessment Protocols (RAPs) that are part of the Resident Assessment Instrument (RAI) that is required by regulation. This comprehensive assessment regulation is the foundation of a clinical record documentation system. Nursing facilities will find that adherence to the RAI process will go a long way to assuring compliance at survey time.

5. Survey Procedures

CMS has developed evaluative questions to assist in determining whether the regulations are being met. In each section of the regulations, surveyors are provided with investigative tools to determine if the facility is in compliance.

These questions can be used by the facility in several productive ways for survey preparation and improving care, such as:

- Staff training in care delivery and documentation.
- Resident/family satisfaction questionnaires.

6. Documentation Guidelines

Each documentation guideline is specific for IDT input, orders, care plans and progress notes. The twelve regulatory domains for Quality of Care are addressed in a chapter of this book.

Activities of Daily Living
Communication and Vision
Pressure Sores
Urinary Incontinence
Range of Motion
Mental and Psychosocial Functioning
Feeding Tubes
Accidents
Nutrition
Hydration
Psychotropic Drugs
Restraints

Although there is no specific section of the federal regulations that addresses pain management, the surveyor procedures include investigative questions to assess whether pain could be an issue, such as in activities of daily living (ADLs), pressure ulcers or incontinence management.

7. Care Delivery System

The federal regulations for comprehensive assessment that require the RAI/MDS are a framework for documentation. The RAI is designed to assist facilities with identification of the resident's strengths, weaknesses, risk factors for deterioration and potential for improvement.

Introduction

The RAP's are tools for staff to assess resident needs and make decisions for care planning. When RAP's are triggered, the interdisciplinary team develops an appropriate care plan with interventions to prevent deterioration and/or promote restoration of deficits, within the limits of:

- a resident's right to refuse treatment, and
- recognized pathology and the normal aging process.

The progress notes of health care professionals are an evaluation of the response of the resident to care plan interventions and the progress, regress or maintenance in terms of the established care plan goals. Progress notes document the outcomes of care and are evidence of the quality of care provided to residents.

Each step in care delivery has a companion documentation step:

Resident Care	**Documentation**
Assessment	Minimum Data Set MDS/RAI
Identify Problems	Resident Assessment Protocols
Goal Setting	Resident Care Plan
Implementation	Medication/Treatment/ ADL Flow Sheets, etc

Documentation is more than a paperwork exercise. It is one piece of the health care delivery system. Just as a jig saw puzzle must have all pieces present in order for the picture to be complete, documentation is an essential piece of health care delivery.

CARE PLANS

The care plan flows from the problems, needs and strengths identified by resident assessment. Completion of the MDS and working the RAP's are tools to identify resident needs and set realistic, attainable goals that are resident-oriented. Unmet needs or unidentified problems can result in a decline in a resident's condition and undesired outcomes of care.

A coordinated interdisciplinary team (IDT) is essential for meeting all resident's needs and achieving good outcomes of care. Just as in playing team sports, such as, baseball, basketball or football, all players must perform their assigned tasks. If one player does not perform, the entire team fails.

Do not underestimate the potential for success that results from resident and family involvement in care planning. Approach the care plan process from a resident-centered viewpoint that allows resident and family participation and choices. The result will not only support and empower the residents to achieve optimal outcomes of care, but also promote resident and family satisfaction which is a measurement of quality of care.

1. Federal Regulations

Section 483.20(k) addresses several issues relating to comprehensive care plans, such as, the structure of the care plan content, time-frame for development and review, input from an interdisciplinary team (IDT) and the participation of the resident and family or legal representative.

Care Plans

The regulations for care plans state:

(1) ***The facility must develop a comprehensive care plan for each resident that includes measurable objectives and timetables to meet a resident's medical, nursing, and mental and psychosocial needs that are identified in the comprehensive assessment. The care plan must describe the following:***

- ***(i)*** ***The services that are to be furnished to attain or maintain the resident's highest practicable physical, mental, and psychosocial well-being as required under §483.25 (Quality of Care); and***

- ***(ii)*** ***Any services that would otherwise be required under §483.25 Quality of Care but are not provided due to the resident's exercise of rights under §483.10 Resident Rights, including the right to refuse treatment under 483.10(b)(4).***

(2) ***A comprehensive care plan must be--***

- ***(i)*** ***Developed within 7 days after the completion of the comprehensive assessment;***

- ***(ii)*** ***Prepared by an interdisciplinary team, that includes the attending physician, a registered nurse with responsibility for the resident, and other appropriate staff in disciplines as determined by the resident's needs, and, to the extent practicable, the participation of the resident, the resident's family or the resident's legal representative; and***

- ***(iii)*** ***Periodically reviewed and revised by a team of qualified persons after each assessment.***

2. Surveyor Guidance for Care Plans

The following guidance to surveyors has been published by CMS for evaluating the facility's compliance with federal regulations Section 483.20(k) Comprehensive Care Plans.

An interdisciplinary team, in conjunction with the resident, resident's family, surrogate, or representative, as appropriate, should develop quantifiable objectives for the highest level of functioning the resident may be expected to attain, based on the comprehensive assessment.

The interdisciplinary team should show evidence in the RAP summary or clinical record of the following:

- The resident's status in triggered RAP areas;
- The facility's rationale for deciding whether to proceed with care planning; and
- Evidence that the facility considered the development of care planning interventions for all RAPs triggered by the MDS.

The care plan must reflect intermediate steps for each outcome objective if identification of those steps will enhance the resident's ability to meet his/her objectives. Facility staff will use these objectives to monitor resident progress. Facilities may, for some residents, need to prioritize their care plan interventions. This should be noted in the clinical record or on the plan or care.

In some cases, a resident may wish to refuse certain services or treatments that professional staff believe may be indicated to assist the resident in reaching his or her highest practicable level of well-being. Desires of the resident should be documented in the clinical record . . . While federal regulations affirm the resident's right to participate in care planning and to refuse treatment, the regulations do not create the right for a resident, legal surrogate or representative to demand that the facility use specific medical intervention or treatment that the facility deems inappropriate. Statutory requirements hold the facility ultimately accountable for the resident's care and safety, including clinical decisions.

When a resident's condition changes or the care plan goals are not met, the care plan is revised with adjusted and new interventions. Usually this is done quarterly during the regular review of MDS information. But it must be done at any time in-between, if the goals of the care plan are not met or the resident's condition changes.

Examples of care plan goals not being met can include:

- Falls or injuries,
- Unplanned weight loss,
- Recurrent urinary tract infections, such as, two or more within 6 months),
- Decrease in range of motion or the development of joint contractures.

3. Surveyor Guidance for Interdisciplinary Team

The following guidance to surveyors has been published by CMS for evaluating the facility's compliance with federal regulations.

The physician must participate as part of the interdisciplinary team, and may arrange with the facility for alternative methods, other than attendance at care planning conferences, of providing his/her input, such as one-on-one discussions and conference calls. . .

The facility has a responsibility to assist residents to participate, e.g., helping residents, and families, legal surrogates or representatives understand the assessment and care planning process; when feasible, holding care planning meetings at the time of day when a resident is functioning best; planning enough time for information exchange and decision making; encouraging a resident's advocate to attend (e.g. family member, friend) if desired by a resident.

"Interdisciplinary" means that health care professionals, as appropriate, will work together to provide the greatest benefit to the resident.

At a minimum, the IDT should include input from:

- the attending physician,
- the licensed nurse responsible for the resident,
- the certified nursing assistant assigned to the resident,
- activity professional,
- social worker and
- dietitian or dietary manager.
- If the resident is receiving restorative therapy, the therapist would also be involved.

The mechanics of how the interdisciplinary team (IDT) meets their responsibility of developing an interdisciplinary care plan is at the discretion of the facility. It may be accomplished by:

- a face-to-face meeting,
- teleconference,
- written communication or
- other methods specified in facility procedures.

In using the resident assessment protocols (RAPs) to develop care plans, several team members will provide input. For example, the Cognitive Loss/Dementia RAP states that this RAP addresses not only the daily living skills of the resident but also their need for meaningful leisure time. Nursing, therapy and activity staffs all may contribute.

IDT input can be accomplished in two ways:

- Each discipline has a clearly identified problem complex written in each care plan, or
- Each discipline contributes causal factors to define the problem statements, goals unique to their discipline, and interventions they plan to implement or recommend.

Participation by the resident or resident's family/legal representative in care planning is essential for success. When setting goals, resident and family cooperation and understanding is needed so all may work toward a common end. The care plan should be resident-oriented and include opportunities for the resident to exercise choice and self-determination, whenever possible.

4. Survey Procedures

During the survey process, a sample of care plans will be reviewed. Surveyors will focus on the unique needs of each resident as identified through the MDS/RAP process. Surveyors will also determine if the care plan is actually carried out as written.

Surveyors will review clinical record documentation to evaluate compliance.

- *Does the care plan address the needs, strengths and preferences identified in the comprehensive resident assessment?*

- *Is the care plan oriented toward preventing avoidable declines in functioning or functional levels? How does the care plan attempt to manage risk factors? Does the care plan build on resident strengths?*

- *Does the care plan reflect standards of current professional practice?*

- *Do treatment objectives have measurable outcomes?*

The surveyors are instructed to:

Corroborate information regarding the resident's goals and wishes for treatment in the plan of care by interviewing residents; especially those identified as refusing treatment.

Determine whether the facility has provided adequate information to the resident so that the resident was able to make an informed choice regarding treatment.

- *If the resident has refused treatment, does the care plan reflect the facility's efforts to find alternative means to address the problem?*

- *Was interdisciplinary expertise utilized to develop a plan to improve the resident's functional abilities? For example, did an occupational therapist design needed adaptive equipment or a speech therapist provide techniques to improve swallowing ability?*

- *Do the dietitian and speech therapist determine, for example, the optimum textures and consistency for the resident's food that provide both a nutritionally adequate diet and effectively use oropharyngeal capabilities of the resident?*

- *Is there evidence of physician involvement in development of the care plan (e.g., presence at care plan meetings, conversations with team members concerning the care plan, conference calls)?*

- *In what ways do staff involve residents and families, surrogates, and/or representatives in care planning? Do staff make an effort to schedule care plan meetings at the best time of the day for residents and their families?*

- *Do facility staff attempt to make the process understandable to the resident/family? Ask residents whether they have brought questions or concerns about their care to th attention of facility's staff. If so, what happened as a result?*

- *Is the care plan evaluated and revised as the resident's status changes?*

5. Procedures for Care Planning

A plan is developed which outlines the care to be given, the objectives to be accomplished and the professional discipline responsible for each element of care. The care plan is initiated on admission for any immediate needs. Then, the comprehensive care plan is completed seven (7) days following the completion of the resident assessment instrument (RAI).

Periodically, the resident care plan is reviewed, evaluated and updated by the health professionals involved in the care of the resident. At a minimum the plan is reviewed quarterly by the interdisciplinary team and coordinated with each minimum data set (MDS) assessment. The care plan is revised more often if there is a change in the resident's condition or the goals of the care plan are not achieved.

- On admission a resident care plan is started with all known immediate problems and needs for the resident.

- A comprehensive care plan is developed for each resident that includes measurable objectives and timetables to meet a resident's medical, nursing and mental and psychosocial needs that are identified through the comprehensive assessment process and input from the interdisciplinary team (IDT).

- The resident's problems and needs are identified from those triggered by the Minimum Data Set, review of the physician's orders for services to be provided or withheld and input from supplemental assessments of other appropriate staff in disciplines determined by the resident's needs.

- The Resident Care Plan includes input from appropriate members of the interdisciplinary team, the resident, the resident's family or the resident's legal representative.

- Short Term Goals (Intermediate Steps) are identified for each problem in measurable, observable terms. Goals provide a mechanism for evaluating resident progress.

- A realistic time limit in which to accomplish each goal is established. If a problem is of an ongoing nature, indicate "every 3 months" as the time limit or the date of the next schedule care plan review.

- Care to be given (actions and approaches) specify the interventions implemented to accomplish the objective for each problem.

- The professional discipline responsible for each intervention is identified.

- The date that a problem was identified is recorded and should remain the same until the problem is resolved.

- As the resident's condition and capacity changes, the resident care plan is updated. Clearly specify date of additions and deletions to the care plan.

- After each quarterly MDS assessment, the plan is reviewed, evaluated and updated by the all professional personnel involved in the care of the resident. The date of each quarterly review is indicated on the resident care plan.

- When a problem is resolved, a yellow highlighter pen is used to mark through the problem. The word "Resolved" and the date are recorded.

- The care plan is written in ink or generated by computer. The care plan is a part of the resident's health record.

6. Tips for Writing Care Plans

To be meaningful, the care plan must be "user-friendly." Terminology should be used that all staff can understand at all professional levels. The care plan should be concise and to the point.

Be sure that the care plan is easy to read. Leave enough space between each problem or use one page per problem to allow room for updating and additional input. Rewrite or reprint from computer software only as necessary to maintain clarity.

Short term problems are often written on a separate page from the comprehensive care plan. This simplifies using the care plan and often eliminates the need for frequent recopying to maintain a usable care plan free from the clutter of "yellowed out" or resolved problems.

All short term problems, both current and resolved, should be reviewed regularly to determine if there should be a prevention problem identified on the comprehensive care plan. For example, if a resident falls, there should be not only a care plan problem to observe and treat any injuries; but also a care plan problem to prevent further falls with intervention developed based on the post fall assessment.

Describe problems, goals and approaches in language that staff can understand. Clearly state what is to be done. For example, *"Remind resident to use walker when ambulating in hallways"* can be clearly understood. Avoid complicated instructions such as, *"Resident will maintain optimal ambulation within the limits of his disease and strength as evidence by the resident maintaining his ability for ambulation in hallways with the use of assistive devices."*

Simplify care plans to save staff time and increase their understanding of the care to be provided. There is no need to include instructions that are universally understood standards of practice, such as *"answer call bell promptly"*. All call bells should be answered promptly. However, a resident specific instructions, such as, *"place call bell on resident's left side,"* would be an important unique instruction for a particular resident.

Personalize care plans to the resident. One resident may wish to be called by a nickname, but for another a nickname would be undignified. Some residents have customary routines that are very important to them, or special places that they prefer to sit during the day.

PROGRESS NOTES

Progress notes evaluate the resident's response to care plan interventions in measurable terms and describe the progress toward goal achievement. Any discrepancy between what is actually happening and what was care planned is clarified. The assessment, care plan and progress notes must agree in content.

Progress notes in a clinical record are the documentation of outcomes of care. The notes are used to communicate relevant and essential information in a concise manner about the resident's condition as well as to serve as evidence of the care that was provided.

1. Frequency of Progress Notes

Nursing staff must have the ability to identify clinically and/or legally significant events that require narrative documentation. Meaningful and informative progress notes are written by staff as often as the resident's condition warrants.

Daily licensed nurses notes are recorded according to facility policy, such as:

- for the first 72 hours following admission,
- for residents on Medicare to demonstrate skilled nursing care,

- when a resident is in critical condition, or
- when the resident's condition changes, until 24 hours after the symptoms have resolved.

On a regular basis, summary nurses' progress notes are written by licensed nurses for each resident specific to the resident's needs, the resident care plan and the resident's response to care and treatment. The frequency of summary narrative nursing notes by the licensed nurse are specified by State regulations, usually weekly or monthly.

Nursing summary notes evaluate:

- the progress or lack of progress toward the goals set in the care plan,
- the resident's response to care and treatment, and
- new problems that occurred during the period of time the summary covers.

Establish a schedule for regularly writing summary notes. Spread the work over a period of time and all shifts. Each resident should be evaluated over a twenty-four (24) hour period from the perspective of each nursing shift. The resulting summaries will give a complete picture of the resident's condition over time.

2. Time

All progress notes, except summary notes, should be timed. When looking back at a resident's clinical course, the exact time of occurrence is often important to assess the resident's condition. Time of admission or discharge are legal entries that determine precisely when the resident became the responsibility of the facility.

The following contacts with physicians should have time recorded as part of the documentation:

- Telephone or verbal orders received from physicians,
- Noting orders to verify implementation,
- Physician notification of admission of a resident,
- Physician notification of changes in the resident's condition, or
- Notification of family or responsible person of changes in the resident's condition should also include time.

3. Content of Progress Notes

Progress notes document the results of the care plan. On a regular basis, progress notes are written that assess the resident's progress, regress or maintenance toward the goals specified in the care plan.

Descriptions should be specific to the resident's condition. Observe for objective findings. Describe what is seen. If the resident makes subjective statements, record them as *"Resident states that . . ."*

Do not use terms that are nonspecific. Terms such as *"usually, frequently, at times or occasionally"* are not measurable. Measurable recording is the documentation of the number of times, how many times, and what time an event occurred.

Progress notes must be concise. Do not repeat a description of the care plan or repeat the physician orders. Do not repeat information contained elsewhere in the clinical record unless the information is needed for clarity.

4. Steps for Writing Summary Progress Notes

Summary nursing progress notes are written on a regular basis as mandated by state regulations, weekly, monthly or quarterly. Before writing a progress note follow these steps:

- Observe the resident's response to nursing interventions.
- Discuss the resident with other staff to identify any changes in condition.
- Review physician orders for new or discontinued orders that may influence the resident's level of care.
- Review PRN medications and treatments to identify increased need for staff intervention.
- Review flow sheets, e.g. ADL flow sheets, weight record, activity attendance logs, behavioral monitoring records, etc., to identify subtle changes in the resident's condition.
- Review previous progress notes to evaluate if resident has changed or short term problems have developed.
- Update the care plan if there is a change in the resident's condition.

5. Flow Sheets

Flow sheets are used to document resident information to be compared over a period of time. Such flow sheets may include:

Bowel/Bladder Retraining
Incontinence Diaries
Pressure Ulcer Progress

Diabetic Monitoring
Enteral Nourishment
Intake and Output
Neurological Signs
Parenteral Fluids
Vital Signs
Weights

Flow sheets enable health professional to record data in a quick and efficient manner. Also, when evaluating the resident's condition, data can be easily found and compared. Use flow sheets to track resident conditions that need comparisons over time.

6. Survey Procedures

Surveyors will review clinical records to determine:

- *How did the resident respond or adjust to care plan interventions?*
- *What is the resident's interactions with staff and other residents?*
- *What is the resident doing now that he/she did not do in the past?*
- *Did an intervention not produce the anticipated result?*
- *Record the degree of success or lack of success in attaining a specific goal.*
- *How has the resident changed since the care plan was written? Are there any new or short term goals?*
- *What actions have been taken to resolve problems and how has the resident responded?*

ACTIVITIES OF DAILY LIVING

The need for supervision or total care of activities of daily living (ADLs) is commonly a primary reason for a resident's continuing stay in a nursing facility. Residents' needs will fall into two categories: restorative and maintenance.

The Resident Assessment Protocol (RAP) for Activities of Daily Living triggers residents with a restorative potential. Assessment and referrals are made to identify any reversible causes of functional decline. For these residents, care plans are developed for rehabilitation and strengthening programs.

The RAP for Activities of Daily Living also includes a maintenance trigger for residents who lack cognitive skills. The Resident Assessment Protocol (RAP) for cognitive deficit recommends a supportive environment to maintain a resident's ADL skills. For these residents nursing care is provided to ensure that ADL status does not decline and that complications are prevented. Complications or poor outcomes of care could be the development or increase of contractures and presence of pressure ulcers.

The RAP for ADL suggests that confounding problems be assessed such as: delirium, persistent mood problems, daily behavior problems, decline in mood or behavior, unstable or acute health problems and the use of psychoactive medications.

The care provided to resident with ADL need includes steps to restore or maintain their abilities. Some of the steps taken can include:

- maintain self-sufficiency of ADLs, utilizing programs of task segmentation, verbal cuing and restorative programs to maintain functioning with fewer supports;

- avoid or delay additional loss of independence by identifying reversible causes of functional decline.

When completing the quarterly MDS be alerted to the MDS/RAI definitions of **"significant change."** Changes in scoring of ADL functions from the previous quarter may signal that a new MDS is required. A significant change assessment is appropriate if there is a consistent pattern of changes, with either two or more areas of decline, or two or more areas of improvement. Significant change reassessments are not required for minor or temporary variations in resident status.

1. Federal Regulations

Section 483.25(a) addresses the need for restoration or maintenance of a resident's abilities to perform activities of daily living.

(a) *Activities of daily living.*

Based on the comprehensive assessment of a resident, the facility must ensure that--

(1) A resident's abilities in activities of daily living do not diminish unless circumstances of the individual's clinical condition demonstrate that diminution was unavoidable. This includes the resident's ability to--

(i) Bathe, dress, and groom;

(ii) Transfer and ambulate;

(iii) Toilet;

(iv) Eat; . . .

(2) ***A resident is given the appropriate treatment and services to maintain or improve his or her abilities specified in paragraph (a) (1) of this section; and***

(3) ***A resident who is unable to carry out activities of daily living receives the necessary services to maintain good nutrition, grooming, and personal and oral hygiene.***

The intent of this regulation is to ensure that a resident's abilities in ADLs do not deteriorate unless the deterioration is unavoidable. Conditions which may demonstrate unavoidable diminution in ADLs may be:

- the progression of the resident's disease,
- the onset of a physical or mental disability, or
- the resident's/representative's refusal of care and treatment in spite of aggressive efforts to counsel and offer alternatives.

2. Quality Measures/Indicators

The following quality measures/indicators are calculated based on data submitted on the MDS. Surveyors will review these measures before visiting the facility to identify focus areas for review.

8.1 Residents who have moderate to severe pain

9.1 Residents whose need for help with daily activities has increased (Bed mobility, transfer, eating and toileting are the daily activities used to calculate this indicator)

9.2 Residents who spend most of their time in a bed or in a chair

9.3 Residents whose ability to move in and around their room got worse

11.2 Prevalence of little or no activity

3. Definitions

The survey guidance provides the following definitions for ADL functions.

Bathing *how the resident takes full-body bath, sponge bath, and transfers in/out of tub or shower.*

Dressing *how resident puts on, fastens and takes off all items of clothing, including donning or removing prosthesis.*

Grooming *how a resident maintains personal hygiene, including preparatory activities, combing hair, brushing teeth, shaving, applying makeup, washing/drying face, hands and perineum.*

Oral hygiene *maintaining the mouth in a clean and intact condition and treating oral pathology such as ulcers of the mucosa. Services to maintain oral hygiene may include brushing the teeth, cleaning dentures, cleaning the mouth and tongue either by assisting the resident with a mouth wash or by manual cleaning with a gauze sponge; and application of medication as prescribed.*

Transfer *how a resident moves between two surfaces, to and from bed, chair, wheelchair to standing position. (Excludes to and from bath/toilet)*

Ambulation *how resident moves between locations in his/her room and adjacent corridor on same floor. If in*

wheelchair, self-sufficiency once in chair.

Toileting *how the resident uses the toilet room (or commode, bedpan, urinal); transfers on/off the toilet, cleanses self, changes pad, manages ostomy/catheter, adjusts clothes.*

Eating *how resident ingests and drinks (regardless of self-feeding skill).*

4. Survey Procedures

The survey procedures instruct the surveyor to sample resident charts to determine that decline in ADL skills has not occurred and that the resident is functioning at the highest practicable level. This includes pain relief and control especially when it is causing a decline or a decrease in the quality of life of the resident.

The survey team will look for a pattern of deterioration in ADLs, such as a number of residents who have deteriorated in more than one ADL or a number of residents who have deteriorated in only one ADL, for example, a number of residents entering the facility continent and now are incontinent.

- *If the resident's abilities . . . have been maintained, what evidence is there that the resident could have improved if appropriate treatment/services were provided?*
- *Are there physical and psychosocial deficits that could affect improvement in functional abilities?*
- *Was the care plan driven by resident strengths identified in the comprehensive assessment?*
- *Was the care plan consistently implemented?*

- *What changes were made in treatment if the resident failed to progress or when initial rehabilitation goals were achieved, but additional progress might have been possible?*

The survey procedures for bathing, dressing and grooming instruct surveyors to sample resident charts to determine:

- *Whether the resident's ability for ADL performance has changed since admission, or over the past 12 months.*

- *Whether the resident's ability to bathe, dress/groom has improved, declined or stayed same.*

- *Whether any deterioration or lack of improvement was avoidable or unavoidable.*

- *Identify if resident triggers RAPs for ADL functional/rehabilitation potential.*

- *What risk factors for decline of bathing, dressing, and/or grooming abilities did the facility identify?*

- *What care did the resident receive to address unique needs to maintain his/her bathing, dressing, and/or grooming abilities (e.g., resident needs a button hook to button his shirt; staff teaches the resident how to use it; staff provides resident with dementia with cues that allow him/her to dress his or herself)?*

- *Were objectives of the care plan periodically evaluated, and if were not met, were alternative approaches developed to encourage maintenance of bathing, dressing, and/or grooming abilities (e.g., resident now unable to button dress, even with encouragement; will ask family if we may use velcro in place of buttons so resident can continue to dress herself)?*

The survey procedures for transfer and ambulation instruct surveyors to sample resident charts to determine:

- *If the resident's transferring and ambulating abilities have declined, what evidence is there that the decline was unavoidable?*

- *What risk factors for decline of transferring or ambulating abilities did the facility identify (e.g., necrotic area of foot ulcer becoming larger, postural hypotension?*

- *What care did the resident receive to address risk factors and unique needs to maintain transferring or ambulating abilities (e.g., a transfer board is provided to maintain ability to transfer from bed to wheelchair and staff teaches the resident how to use it)?*

- *What evidence is there that sufficient staff time and assistance are provided to maintain transferring and ambulating abilities?*

- *Has resident been involved in activities that enhance mobility skills?*

- *Identify if resident triggers RAPS for ADL functional/rehabilitation potential, psycho-social well-being or moods state and the RAPs are followed.*

- *Were individual objectives of the plan of care periodically evaluated, and if goals were not met, were alternative approaches developed to encourage maintenance of transferring and ambulation abilities (e.g., resident remains unsteady when using a cane, returns to walker, with staff encouraging the walker's consistent use)?*

The survey procedures for toileting instruct surveyors to sample resident charts to determine:

- *If the resident's toilet use abilities have declined, what evidence is there that the decline was unavoidable?*

- *What risk factors for the decline of toilet use abilities did the facility identify (e.g., severe arthritis in hands makes use of toilet paper difficult)?*

- *What care did resident receive to address risk factors and unique needs to maintain toilet use abilities (e.g., assistive devices to maintain ability to use the toilet such as using a removable elevated toilet seat or wall grab bar to facilitate rising from seated position to standing position?*

- *Is there sufficient staff time and assistance provided to maintain toilet use abilities (e.g., allowing residents enough time to use the toilet independently or with limited assistance)?*

- *Were individual objectives of the plan of care periodically evaluated, and if objectives were not met, were alternative approaches developed to encourage maintaining toilet use abilities (e.g., if resident has not increased sitting stability, seek occupational therapy consult to determine the need for therapy to increase sitting balance, ability to transfer safely and manipulate clothing during the toileting process. For residents with dementia, remind periodically to use the toilet)?*

- *Identify if resident triggers RAPS for ADL functional/ rehabilitation potential or urinary incontinence.*

The survey procedures for eating instruct surveyors to sample resident charts to determine:

- *If a resident's eating abilities declined, is there any evidence the decline was avoidable or unavoidable?*

- *What risk factors for decline of eating skills did the facility identify?*

  -- *A decrease in the ability to chew and swallow food,*
  -- *Deficit in neurological and muscular status necessary for moving food onto a utensil and into the mouth,*
  -- *Oral health status affecting eating ability, or*
  -- *Depression or confused mental state.*

- *What care did the resident receive to address unique needs to maintain eating abilities?*

  -- *Assistive devices to improve resident's grasp or coordination,*
  -- *Seating arrangements to improve sociability, or*
  -- *Seating in a calm, quiet setting for residents with dementia.*

- *Is there sufficient staff time and assistance provided to maintain eating abilities (e.g., allowing residents enough time to eat independently or with limited assistance)?*

- *Identify if resident triggers RAPs for ADL functional/rehabilitation potential, feeding tubes, and dehydration/fluid maintenance and the RAPs were used to assess causal reasons for decline, potential for decline or lack of improvement.*

- *Were individual objectives of the plan of care periodically evaluated, and if the objectives were not met, were alternative approaches developed to encourage maintaining eating abilities?*

5. Documentation Guidelines for Activity of Daily Living

IDT Input: Nursing, restorative therapy, dietary, activity, social service

Orders: Limitations on weight bearing, activity
Requirement for bed rest
Exercise: ROM, strengthening, balance
Restorative Programs: Eating, walking, dressing
Referral to physical or occupational therapist, psychiatric consult
Pain medication

Care Plan: Rehabilitative goals of several types can be considered:

Restorative Goals

- To restore function to maximum self-sufficiency in the area indicated
- To replace hands-on assistance with a program of task segmentation and verbal cuing
- To restore abilities to a level that allows the resident to function with fewer supports
- To shorten the time required for providing assistance
- To expand the amount of space in which self-sufficiency can be practiced

Maintenance Goals

- To avoid or delay additional loss of independence
- To maintain functional abilities at the same level within the limits of the residents disease process

Approaches and Interventions:

- Amount of staff time and assistance to be provided for ROM, turning or positioning, transfer-ring, ambulating, dressing, and feeding
- Residents who have problems with memory, attention or thinking may benefit from task segmentation of ADLs
- Steps to promote independence in ADL skills, such as cuing, verbal encouragement, scheduling, family involvement
- Special appliances used or needed to assist resident, such as brace, orthopedic footwear, walker/cane, long-handled brush, adaptive eating tools
- Unique needs for resident to maintain his/her ADL skills, removal or modification of environmental barriers or use of physical restraints
- Pain relief and/or control if contributing to decline in ADL skills
- Exercise and restorative programs
- Activity programs, group exercise, movement classes, grooming
- Alternate approaches to maintain ADL skills if objectives have not been meet

Progress Notes:

Bathing, Dressing, Grooming:

- Describe progress, maintenance or regress in resident's ability to bathe, dress or groom self
- Identify any risk factors for decline in ADL skills. Care that is unique to resident needs to maintain bathing, dressing and grooming and amount of staff involvement
- Alternative approaches for bathing, dressing and

grooming when goals have not been met
- Special appliances used to assist resident

Transfer:
- Amount of help provided by the resident, ability to move extremities and the need for assistance
- Risk factors influencing ability to transfer, e.g., foot ulcers, postural hypotension, motivation
- Unique assistance problems, e.g. transfer board, teaching, multiple person assistance
- Special appliances used to assist resident

Locomotion:
- Describe ability to walk once in a standing position. How far can the resident walk? Quality of ambulation?
- Risk factors that impede ambulation, such as pain, motivation, weakness
- Weight bearing limitations, endurance, strength and balance
- Use of a wheelchair, self sufficiency in propelling
- Need for assistance or supportive devices. Ability to use devices

Toileting:
- Ability to use the toilet, assistance with clothing, reminding resident
- Unique needs and assistive devices used, use of urinal
- Physical difficulties, e.g., arthritis, confusion, pain
- Cuing and schedule for maintenance of continence, results of scheduled toileting
- Risk factors such as infections, stress, mentation, lack of motivation

Eating:

- Ability to feed oneself and drink fluids, need for cueing, verbal encouragement
- Assistance provided, ability to handle utensils, special arrangement of food, seating
- Motivation in eating, attention span
- Acceptance of supplemental nourishments
- Difficulty in chewing/swallowing
- Meal environment, socialization at mealtimes

6. Documentation Guidelines for Oral Hygiene

IDT Input: Nursing, social service, dentist, dental hygienist

Orders: Referral to dentist or dental hygienist
Medications and treatments

Care Plan: Interventions for oral hygiene, what tasks performed by resident or by staff

Observation for signs and symptoms of mouth problems

Progress Notes:

- Observation that the mouth cleanliness, presence of oral pathology such as ulcers of the mucosa
- Resident ability to brush teeth, clean dentures, cleaning of oral cavity by use of mouth wash or swabs

COMMUNICATIONS AND VISION

How well a resident understands others can directly influence his or her adjustment to the nursing facility. Hearing loss can result in withdrawal and social isolation. The ability to make one's needs known and to express ideas is a common problem for nursing facility residents, resulting in frustration and the potential for behavioral problems.

The facility may need to make environmental modifications to enhance the resident's self-sufficiency. For example, it may be beneficial to make large print signs marking rooms, special reading lights, large numbers on telephone or clock.

The resident's plan for leisure activities should include programs adapted to the resident's communication, hearing and visual needs. Social services or facility staff assist residents in accessing vision and hearing services. Care plans include referrals to health care professionals, and the need for assistive devices to maintain vision and hearing.

1. Federal Regulations

Section 483.25(a)(1)(v) addresses the need for restoration or maintenance of a resident's abilities to use speech, language or other functional communication systems and Section 483.26(b) for vision and hearing.

(a) *Activities of daily living.*

Based on the comprehensive assessment of a resident, the facility must ensure that--

(1) ***A resident's abilities in activities of daily living do not diminish unless circumstances of the individual's clinical condition demonstrate that diminution was unavoidable. This includes the resident's ability to . . .***

(v) ***Use speech, language, or other functional communication system.***

(b) *Vision and hearing.*

To ensure that residents receive proper treatment and assistive devices to maintain vision and hearing abilities, the facility must, if necessary, assist the resident--

(1) ***In making appointments, and***

(2) ***By arranging for transportation to and from the office of a practitioner specializing in the treatment of vision or hearing impairment or the office of a professional specializing in the provision of vision or hearing assistive devices.***

The intent of this regulation is to require a facility to assist residents in gaining access to vision and hearing services by making appointments and arranging for transportation, and assistance with the use of any devise needed to maintain vision and hearing.

2. Definitions

The surveyor guidance provides the following

definitions for assistive devices:

Assistive Devices

Assistive devices to maintain vision include glasses, contact lenses, and magnifying glasses. Assistive devices to maintain hearing include hearing aids.

Speech, Language or Other Functional Communications Systems

The ability to effectively communicate requests, needs, opinions, and urgent problems; to express emotion, to listen to others, and to participate in social conversation whether in speech, writing, gesture or a combination of these (e.g., a communication board or electronic augmentative communication device.)

This requirement does not mean that the facility must provide refractions, glasses, contact lenses, conduct comprehensive audiological evaluations (although screening is a part of the required assessment in Section 483.20(b)) or provide hearing aids.

The facility's responsibility is to assist residents and their families in locating and utilizing any available resources (e.g., Medicare or Medicaid program payment, local health organizations offering items and services which are available free to the community). Often the responsibility of making appointments and arranging transportation is assumed by the social service department.

3. Survey Procedures

The survey procedures instruct the surveyor to sample resident charts to determine that decline in communication skills have not occurred and that the resident is functioning at the highest practicable level.

Communications and Vision

The surveyor procedures instruct the surveyor to determine for each resident, if resident's ability to communicate has declined, improved or stayed the same and whether any deterioration or lack of improvement was avoidable or unavoidable.

- *Identify if resident triggers RAPs for communication, psychosocial well-being, mood state, and visual function, and if the RAPs were used to assess causal factors for decline, potential for decline or lack of improvement.*

- *What risk factors for decline of communication ability did the facility identify and how did they address them (e.g., dysarthria, poor fitting dentures, few visitors, poor relationships with staff, Alzheimer's disease)?*

- *Has the resident received audiologic and vision evaluation? If not, did the resident refuse such services?*

- *What unique resident needs and risk factors did the facility identify (e.g., does the resident have specific difficulties in transmitting messages, comprehending messages, and/or using a variety of communication skills such as questions and commands; does the resident receive evaluation and training in the use of assistive devices to increase and/or maintain writing skills)?*

- *What care does the resident receive to improve communication abilities (e.g., nurse aides communicate in writing with deaf residents or residents with severe hearing problems; practice exercises with residents receiving speech-language pathology services; increase number of resident's communication opportunities; non-verbal means of communication; review of the effect of medications on communication ability?*

- *Is there sufficient staff time and assistance provided to maintain communication abilities?*

- *Were individual objectives of the plan of care periodically evaluated, and if the objectives were not met, were alternative approaches developed to encourage maintenance of communication abilities (e.g., if drill-oriented therapy is frustrating the resident, a less didactic approach should be attempted)?*

- *If the resident's speech, language and other communication abilities have been maintained, what evidence is there that the resident could have improved if appropriate treatment and services were provided?*

- *Are there physical and psychosocial deficits that could affect improvement of functional abilities?*

- *Was the care plan driven by resident strengths identified in the comprehensive assessment?*

- *Was the care plan consistently implemented?*

- *What changes were made in treatment if the resident failed to progress or when initial rehabilitation goals were achieved, but additional progress might have been possible?*

The surveyor procedures instruct the surveyor to determine if the residents receive proper treatment and assistive devices to maintain <u>vision and hearing</u> abilities.

- *Identify if resident triggers RAPs for visual function, and communication. Consider whether the RAPs were used to assess causal factors for decline, potential for decline or lack of improvement.*

- *If the resident needs, and/or requests and does not have vision and/or hearing assistive devices, what has the facility done to assist the resident in making appointments and obtaining transportation to obtain these services?*

- *If the resident has assistive devices but is not using them, why not (e.g., are repairs or batteries needed)?*

4. Documentation Guidelines for Communications

IDT Input: Nursing, social services, activity, audiologist, speech-language pathologist.

Orders: Referral to audiologist or speech-language pathologist
Hygienic procedures, such as removal of ear wax

Care Plan: Use of hearing appliances and communication aids
Methods of communication, special techniques
Referrals to other health care professionals
Need for staff involvement and restorative programs
Appropriate activity programs for the hearing impaired

Progress Notes:

- Evaluation of use of hearing aide
- Special techniques for communication: e.g., need to speak on good side, communicate in simple ideas
- Ability to communicate requests, opinions, urgent problems and social conversations
- Ability to express emotions, to listen to others and to participate in social conversation
- Method of communication in speech, writing, sign language

- Risks that complicate ability to communicate.
- Psychosocial problems, such as motivation or state of mind affecting communication.

5. Documentation Guidelines for Visual Function

IDT Input: Nursing, social services, activity, ophthalmologist, optometrist

Orders: Referral to ophthalmologist or optometrist
Medications for eye problems
Treatments for eye problems

Care Plan: Use of visual appliances
Environmental modifications
Referrals to health professionals
Medications and treatments
Need for staff involvement and assistance
Appropriate activity programs for the visually impaired

Progress Notes:

- Resident's need for glasses for activities of daily living or special arrangements to facilitate self-performance of ADL
- Ability to use special appliances, such as magnifying glass for reading
- Adaptation to special room arrangements to facilitate mobility or ensure safety
- Amount of assistance provided due to visual deficiency
- Observations for symptoms of acute eye conditions, e.g., eye pain, blurry vision, double vision, and sudden loss of vision, discharge from eye
- Participation in activity pursuits within the limitations of decreased vision

PRESSURE SORES (ULCERS)

The development of a pressure ulcer is a serious clinical complication. Many are preventable with good nursing care. However, others may be unavoidable or difficult to heal due to diabetes, peripheral vascular disease or terminal disease process. For newly admitted residents either at risk or with a pressure ulcer, the staff is expected to assess and provide appropriate care from the day of admission.

On admission, the first step in prevention is to identify the resident at risk of developing pressure ulcers. This is followed by immediate care planning with appropriate individualized interventions to prevent skin breakdown. At least daily, staff should remain alert to potential changes in the skin condition and should evaluate and document when there are identified changes.

1. Federal Regulations

Section 483.25(c) addresses the need for prevention of pressure sores. Although the regulatory language refers to pressure **"sores"**, the nomenclature widely accepted presently refers to pressure **"ulcers"**, and the guidance provide in the regulations refers to pressure **"ulcers"**.

(c) ***Pressure sores.***

Based on the comprehensive assessment of a resident, the facility must ensure that--

Pressure Sores (Ulcers)

(1) ***A resident who enters the facility without pressure sores does not develop pressure sores unless the individual's clinical condition demonstrates that they were unavoidable; and***

(2) ***A resident having pressure sores receives necessary treatment and services to promote healing, prevent infection and prevent new sores from developing.***

The intent of this regulation is that the resident does not develop a pressure ulcer unless clinically unavoidable and that the facility provides care and services to:

- Promote the prevention of pressure ulcer development;
- Promote the healing of pressure ulcers that are present (including prevention of infection to the extent possible); and
- Prevent development of additional pressure ulcers.

2. Quality Measures/Indicators

The following quality measures/indicators are calculated based on data submitted on the MDS. Surveyors will review these measures before visiting the facility to identify focus areas for review.

12.1 High-risk residents with pressure ulcers

12.2 Low-risk residents with pressure ulcers

3. Definitions

The surveyor guidance provides the following definitions:

Pressure Ulcer *A pressure ulcer is any lesion caused by unrelieved pressure that results in damage to the underlying tissue(s). Although friction and shear are not primary causes of pressure ulcers, friction and shear are important contributing factors to the development of pressure ulcers.*

Avoidable *A pressure ulcer developed and that the facility did not do one or more of the following: evaluate the resident's clinical condition and pressure ulcer risk factors; define and implement interventions that are consistent with resident needs, resident goals, and recognized standards of practice; monitor and evaluate the impact of the interventions; or revise the interventions as appropriate.*

Unavoidable *A pressure ulcer developed even though the facility had evaluated the resident's clinical condition and pressure ulcer risk factors; defined and implemented interventions that are consistent with resident needs, goals, and recognized standards of practice; monitored and evaluated the impact of the interventions; and revised the approaches as appropriate.*

Colonized *Refers to the presence of bacteria on the surface or in the tissue of a wound without the signs and symptoms of an infection.*

Infected *Refers to the presence of micro-organisms in sufficient quantity to overwhelm the defenses of viable tissues and produce the signs and symptoms of infection.*

Eschar *A thick, leathery, frequently black or brown in color, necrotic (dead) or devitalized tissue that* *has lost its usual physical properties and biological activity. Eschar may be loose or firmly adhered to the wound.*

Slough *Necrotic/avascular tissue in the process of separating from the viable portions of the body and is usually light colored, soft, moist, and stringy (at times).*

Exudate *Any fluid that has been forced out of the tissues or its capillaries because of inflammation or injury. It may contain serum, cellular debris, bacteria and leukocytes.* ***Purulent*** *exudate/drainage/discharge is any product of inflammation that contains pus (e.g., leukocytes, bacteria, and liquefied necrotic debris).* ***Serous*** *drainage or exudates is watery, clear, or slightly yellow/tan/pink fluid that has separated from the blood and presents as drainage.*

Friction *The mechanical force exerted on skin that is dragged across any surface.*

Shearing *The interaction of both gravity and friction against the surface of the skin. Friction is always present when shear force is present. Shear occurs when layers of skin rub against each other or when the skin remains stationary and the underlying tissue moves and stretches and angulates or tears the underlying capillaries and blood vessels causing tissue damage.*

Granulation *Pink-red moist tissue that fills an open wound, when it starts to heal. It contains new blood vessels, collagen, fibroblasts, and inflammatory cells.*

NOTE: *Tunnel / Sinus Tract / Undermining"- Tunnel and sinus tract are often used interchangeably.*

Tunneling *A passageway of tissue destruction under the skin surface that has an opening at the skin level from the edge of the wound.*

Sinus tract *A cavity or channel underlying a wound that involves an area larger than the visible surface of the wound.*

Undermining *The destruction of tissue or ulceration extending under the skin edges (margins) so that the pressure ulcer is larger at its base than at the skin surface. Undermining often develops from shearing forces and is differentiated from tunneling by the larger extent of the wound edge involved in undermining and the absence of a channel or tract extending from the pressure ulcer under the adjacent intact skin.*

The surveyor guidance outlines definitions for the stages of pressure ulcers. The staging system is one method of summarizing certain characteristics of pressure ulcers, including the extent of tissue damage. This is the system used within the MDS/RAI. The definitions for the stages of pressure ulcers identified below are from the NPUAP (National Pressure Ulcer Advisory Panel) and used in the CMS SOM Appendix PP Surveyor Guidelines.

Stage I *An observable, pressure-related alteration of intact skin, whose indicators as compared to an adjacent or opposite area on the body may include changes in one or more of the following parameters:*

- *Skin temperature (warmth or coolness);*
- *Tissue consistency (firm or boggy);*
- *Sensation (pain, itching); and/or*
- *A defined area of persistent redness in lightly pigmented skin, whereas in darker skin tones, the ulcer may appear with persistent red, blue, or purple hues.*

Stage II *Partial thickness skin loss involving epidermis, dermis, or both. The ulcer is superficial and presents clinically as an abrasion, blister, or shallow crater.*

Stage III *Full thickness skin loss involving damage to, or necrosis of, subcutaneous tissue that may extend down to, but not through, underlying fascia. The ulcer presents clinically as a deep crater with or without undermining of adjacent tissue.*

Stage IV *Full thickness skin loss with extensive destruction, tissue necrosis, or damage to muscle, bone, or supporting structures (e.g., tendon, joint capsule). Undermining and sinus tracts also may be associated with Stage IV pressure ulcers.*

***NOTE**: If eschar and necrotic tissue are covering and preventing adequate staging of a pressure ulcer, the RAI User's Manual Version 2 instructs the assessor to code the pressure ulcer as a Stage IV. These instructions must be followed for MDS coding purposes until they are revised. Although the AHCPR and NPUAP system for staging pressure ulcers indicates that the presence of eschar precludes accurate staging of the ulcer, the facility must use the RAI directions in order to code the MDS, but not necessarily to render treatment.*

4. Surveyor Guidance

The following are key points from the CMS clinical guidance to surveyors.

A standardized pressure ulcer risk assessment tool should be used to assess a resident's pressure ulcer risks upon admission, weekly for the first four weeks after admission for each resident at risk, then quarterly, or whenever there is a change in cognition or functional ability. Examples of a resident's risk increasing that would require additional evaluation could be due to an acute illness or condition change (e.g., upper respiratory infection, pneumonia, or exacerbation of underlying congestive heart failure).

Some examples of risk factors:

- Impaired/decreased mobility and decreased functional ability;
- Co-morbid conditions, such as end stage renal disease, thyroid disease or diabetes mellitus;
- Drugs such as steroids that may affect wound healing;
- Impaired diffuse or localized blood flow, for example, generalized atherosclerosis or lower extremity arterial insufficiency;
- Resident refusal of some aspects of care and treatment;
- Cognitive impairment;
- Exposure of skin to urinary and fecal incontinence;
- Under nutrition, malnutrition, and hydration deficits; and

- A healed ulcer. The history of a healed pressure ulcer and its stage [if known] is important, since areas of healed Stage III or IV pressure ulcers are more likely to have recurrent breakdown.

While pressure ulcers on the sacrum remain the most common location, pressure ulcers on the heel are occurring more frequently, are difficult to assess and heal, and require early identification of skin compromise over the heel. Pressure ulcers may develop at other sites where pressure has impaired the circulation to the tissue, such as pressure from positioning or use of medical devices.

Three of the more common types of ulcers are pressure, vascular insufficiency/ischemia (venous stasis and arterial ischemic ulcers) and neuropathic. At the time of the assessment, clinicians (physicians, advance practice nurses, physician assistants, and certified wound care specialists, etc.) should document the clinical basis (for example, type of skin injury/ulcer, location, shape, ulcer edges and wound bed, condition of surrounding tissues) for any determination that an ulcer is not pressure-related, especially if the injury/ulcer has characteristics consistent with a pressure ulcer, but is determined not to be one.

It is important that each existing pressure ulcer be identified, whether present on admission or developed after admission, and that factors that influenced its development, the potential for development of additional ulcers or for the deterioration of the pressure ulcer(s) be recognized, assessed and addressed. Any new pressure ulcer suggests a need to reevaluate the adequacy of the plan for preventing pressure ulcers.

When assessing the ulcer itself, it is important to:

- Differentiate the type of ulcer (pressure-related versus non-pressure-related) because interventions may vary depending on the specific type of ulcer;

- Determine the ulcer's stage;
- Describe and monitor the ulcer's characteristics;
- Monitor the progress toward healing and for potential complications;
- Determine if infection is present;
- Assess, treat and monitor pain, if present; and
- Monitor dressings and treatments.

It is important that the facility have a system in place to assure that the protocols for daily monitoring and for periodic documentation of measurements, terminology, frequency of assessment, and documentation are implemented consistently throughout the facility. The amount of observation possible will depend upon the type of dressing that is used, since some dressings are meant to remain in place for several days, according to manufacturers' guidelines.

With each dressing change or at least weekly (and more often when indicated by wound complications or changes in wound characteristics), an evaluation of the pressure ulcer wound should be documented. At a minimum, documentation should include the date observed and:

- Location and staging;
- Size (perpendicular measurements of the greatest extent of length and width of the ulceration), depth; and the presence, location and extent of any undermining or tunneling/sinus tract;
- Exudate, if present: type (such as purulent/serous), color, odor and approximate amount;

- Pain, if present: nature and frequency (e.g., whether episodic or continuous);

- Wound bed: Color and type of tissue/character including evidence of healing (e.g., granulation tissue), or necrosis (slough or eschar); and

- Description of wound edges and surrounding tissue (e.g., rolled edges, redness, hardness/induration, maceration) as appropriate.

Current literature reports that all Stage II, III, and IV pressure ulcers are colonized with bacteria but may not be infected. Wounds may be classified as infected if the signs and symptoms of infection are present and/or a wound culture (obtained in accord with accepted standards, such as sterile tissue aspirate, a "quantitative surface swab" using the Levine technique or semi-quantitative swab) contains 100,000 or greater micro-organisms per gram of tissue. A superficial swab may show the presence of bacteria, but is not a reliable method to identify infection.

5. Survey Procedure

The surveyor procedures instruct the surveyor to sample resident charts for residents at risk of developing pressure sores.

- *Identify if resident triggers RAPs for urinary incontinence, nutritional status, cognitive loss/dementia, psychotropic drugs use, and physical restraints.*

- *Consider whether the RAPs were used to assess causal factors for decline, potential for decline or lack of improvement.*

- *Is aggressive preventive care provided?*

If a dressing change is scheduled during the survey, observe the wound care to determine if the record reflects the current status of the ulcer(s) and note:

- *Characteristics of the wound and surrounding tissues such as presence of granulation tissue, the Stage, presence of exudates, necrotic tissue such as eschar or slough, or evidence of erythema or swelling around the wound;*

- *The form or type of debridement, if used;*

- *Whether treatment and infection control practices reflect current standards of practice; and*

- *Based on location, steps taken to cleanse and protect the wound from likely contamination by urine or fecal incontinence.*

If unable to observe the dressing change due to the dressing protocol, observe the area surrounding the ulcer(s). For ulcers with dressings that are not scheduled to be changed, the surveyor may request that the dressing be removed to observe the wound and surrounding area if other information suggests a possible treatment or assessment problem.

If the resident expresses (or appears to be in) pain related to the ulcer or treatment, determine if the facility:

- *Assessed for pain related to the ulcer, addressed and monitored interventions for effectiveness; and/or*

- *Assessed and took preemptive measures for pain related to dressing changes or other treatments, such as debridement / irrigations, and monitored for effectiveness.*

Pressure Sores (Ulcers)

The surveyors are instructed to review the RAI and other documents such as physician orders, progress notes, nurses' notes, pharmacy or dietary notes regarding the assessment of the resident's overall condition, risk factors and presence of a pressure ulcer(s) to determine if the facility identified the resident at risk and evaluated the factors placing the resident at risk:

- *For a resident who was admitted with an ulcer or who developed one within 1 to 2 days, review the admission documentation regarding the wound site and characteristics at the time of admission, the possibility of underlying tissue damage because of immobility or illness prior to admission, skin condition on or within a day of admission, history of impaired nutrition; and history of previous pressure ulcers; and*

- *For a resident who subsequently developed or has an existing pressure ulcer, review documentation regarding the wound site, characteristics, progress and complications including reassessment if there were no signs of progression towards healing within 2 to 4 weeks.*

In considering the appropriateness of a facility's response to the presence, progression, or deterioration of a pressure ulcer, take into account the resident's condition, complications, time needed to determine the effectiveness of a treatment, and the facility's efforts, where possible, to remove, modify, or stabilize the risk factors and underlying causal factors.

For the resident at risk for developing or who has a pressure ulcer, determine if the facility developed an individualized care plan that addresses prevention, care and treatment of any existing pressure ulcers, including specific interventions, measurable objectives and approximate time frames.

If the facility's care of a specific resident refers to a treatment protocol that contains details of the treatment regimen, the care plan should refer to that protocol. The care plan should clarify any major deviations from, or revisions to, that protocol in a specific resident.

A specific care plan intervention for risk of pressure ulcers is not needed if other components of the care plan address related risks adequately. For example, the risk of skin breakdown posed by fecal/urinary incontinence might be addressed in that part of the care plan that deals with incontinence management.

If the resident refuses or resists staff interventions to reduce risk or treat existing pressure ulcers, determine if the care plan reflects efforts to seek alternatives to address the needs identified in the assessment.

Determine if the staff have been monitoring the resident's response to interventions for prevention and/or treatment and have evaluated and revised the care plan based on the resident's response, outcomes, and needs. Review the record and interview staff for information and/or evidence that:

- *Continuing the current approaches meets the resident's needs, if the resident has experienced recurring pressure ulcers or lack of progression toward healing and staff did not revise the care plan; and*

- *The care plan was revised to modify the prevention strategies and to address the presence and treatment of a newly developed pressure ulcer, for the resident who acquired a new ulcer.*

6. Documentation Guidelines for Pressure Ulcers

IDT Input: Nursing, dietary, physical therapy, physician, wound specialist, infection control

Pressure Sores (Ulcers)

Assessment: Observation of resident's skin integrity on admission

Identify risk for developing a pressure ulcer using a standard risk assessment, such as the Braden Scale. Complete standard risk assessment on the day of admission and then once a week for the next four weeks. Update risk assessment quarterly.

A comprehensive assessment or MDS RAP documentation:

- risk factors,
- pressure points,
- undernutrition and hydration deficits, and
- moisture and the impact of moisture

Clinical justification for the unavoidable development or non-healing/delayed healing or deterioration of a pressure ulcer;

Orders: Treatment to open area
Dressings, frequency of changes
Medications for pain or infection
Pressure reducing devices
Diagnostic lab tests and wound cultures
Infection control precautions
Nutritional supplements
Hydration

Care Plan: **For residents at risk for pressure ulcers:**

- Protective/preventative skin care
- Turning/repositioning, methods to prevent further injury, and frequency of positioning
- Pressure relieving beds/chair pads
- Encourage ambulation/movement and

time out of bed
- Range of motion exercises
- Nutritional supplements
- Pain management to enable mobility

For residents with pressure ulcers:
- Wound care/treatment
- Interventions to promote healing
- Infection control precautions
- Other skin treatment
- Nutritional interventions
- Pain management related to treatment

If a pressure ulcer is not healing, getting larger or there are signs of additional skin breakdown, re-evaluate care plan with alternate interventions

If a pressure ulcer recurs after healing, re-evaluate plan to prevent pressure sores

After a pressure ulcer has healed, develop interventions to prevent further skin breakdown

Progress Notes:

Treatment interventions ordered by physician to prevent skin breakdown,
Nutritional supplements and intake
Evaluation of condition changes of skin, (inspect skin at least once daily)

Routine preventative and restorative care:
- turning and proper positioning
- application of pressure reduction or relief devices
- providing good skin care, such as, keep skin clean, individualized bathing

schedule
- instituting measures to reduce excessive moisture
- providing clean, dry bed linens
- maintaining adequate nutrition
- rehabilitation program

Evaluation of risk factors, such as
- urinary incontinence
- poor nutritional status
- cognitive loss or dementia
- psychotropic drug use
- physical restraints, and
- decreased mobility

Documentation of **risks where the development of pressure ulcers may be unavoidable**
- terminally ill and end stage disease
- poor circulation, due to peripheral vascular disease, etc
- diabetes
- orthopedic casts

Weekly description of open skin or lesions:
- site
- size
- color
- exudate
- odor. and
- stage

Notify the physician when a pressure ulcer first occurs and when a pressure ulcer deteriorates or does not respond to treatment.

Observe for **signs of Infection,**

- if drainage is present: purulent exudate
- peri-wound warmth, swelling, induration or erythema (erythema may not be readily determined in individuals with dark skin pigmentation)
- increasing pain or tenderness around the site or
- delayed wound healing
- Document if a culture was taken and if isolation precautions are necessary

Pain that interferes with movement and/or affects mood

- Pain management associated with treatment and dressing changes

Documentation of resident **refusal or resistance to care**, if applicable

- Alternative offered to address the resident's needs
- Counselling regarding risks

64

URINARY INCONTINENCE

Urinary incontinence is a frequent problem for residents in a nursing facility. Management of incontinence is not only costly and time consuming for staff; but also can lead to serious complications for the resident, such as, skin breakdown and urinary tract infection.

1. Federal Regulations

Section 483.25(d) addresses three issues: the management of incontinence, the use of foley catheters, and the prevention of urinary tract infections.

(d) ***<u>Urinary Incontinence.</u>***

Based on the resident's comprehensive assessment, the facility must ensure that--

(1) ***A resident who enters the facility without an indwelling catheter is not catheterized unless the resident's clinical condition demonstrates that catheterization was necessary; and***

(2) ***A resident who is incontinent of bladder receives appropriate treatment and services to prevent urinary tract infections and to restore as much normal bladder function as possible.***

The intent of this requirement is to ensure that:

- Each resident who is incontinent of urine is identified, assessed and provided appropriate treatment and services to achieve or maintain as much normal urinary function as possible;

- An indwelling catheter is not used unless there is valid medical justification;

- An indwelling catheter for which continuing use is not medically justified is discontinued as soon as clinically warranted;

- Services are provided to restore or improve normal bladder function to the extent possible, after the removal of the catheter; and

- A resident, with or without a catheter, receives the appropriate care and services to prevent infections to the extent possible.

2. Quality Measures/Indicators

The following quality measures/indicators are calculated based on data submitted on the MDS. Surveyors will review these measures before visiting the facility to identify focus areas for review.

5.1 Low-risk residents who lost control of their bowels or bladder

5.2 Residents who have/had a catheter inserted and left in their bladder

5.3 Prevalence of occasional or frequent bladder or bowel incontinence without a toileting plan

5.4 Prevalence of fecal impaction

6.1 Residents with a urinary tract infection

3. Definitions

The surveyor guidance provides the following definitions for assessment of the types of incontinence:

Urge *Characterized by abrupt urgency, frequency, and nocturia (part of the overactive bladder diagnosis). It may be age-related or have neurological causes (e.g., stroke, diabetes mellitus, Parkinson's Disease, multiple sclerosis) or other causes such as bladder infection, urethral irritation, etc. The resident can feel the need to void, but is unable to inhibit voiding long enough to reach and sit on the commode. It is the most common cause of urinary incontinence in elderly persons.*

Stress *Loss of a small amount of urine with physical activity such as coughing, sneezing, laughing, walking stairs or lifting. Urine leakage results from an increase in intra-abdominal pressure on a bladder that is not over distended and is not the result of detrusor contractions. It is the second most common type of urinary incontinence in older women.*

Mixed *combination of urge incontinence and stress incontinence. Many elderly persons (especially women) will experience symptoms of both urge and stress called mixed incontinence.*

Overflow *Occurs when the bladder is distended from urine retention. Symptoms of overflow incontinence may include: weak stream, hesitancy, or inter-*

mittency; dysuria; nocturia; frequency; incomplete voiding; frequent or constant dribbling. Urine retention may result from outlet obstruction (e.g., benign prostatic hypertrophy (BPH), prostate cancer, and urethral stricture), hypotonic bladder (detrusor under activity) or both. Hypotonic bladder may be caused by outlet obstruction, impaired or absent contractility of the bladder (neurogenic bladder) or other causes. Neurogenic bladder may also result from neurological conditions such as diabetes mellitus, spinal cord injury, or pelvic nerve damage from surgery or radiation therapy. In overflow incontinence, post void residual (PVR) volume (the amount of urine remaining in the bladder within 5 to 10 minutes following urination) exceeds 200 milliliters (ml). Normal PVR is usually 50 ml. or less. A PVR of 150 to 200 may suggest a need for retesting to determine if this finding is clinically significant. Overflow incontinence may mimic urge or stress incontinence but is less common than either of those.

Functional *Secondary to factors other than inherently abnormal urinary tract function. It may be related to physical weakness or poor mobility/dexterity (e.g., due to poor eyesight, arthritis, deconditioning, stroke, contracture), cognitive problems (e.g., confusion, dementia, unwillingness to toilet), various medications (e.g., anti-cholinergics, diuretics) or environmental impediments (e.g., excessive distance of the resident from the toilet facilities, poor lighting, low chairs that are difficult to get out of, physical restraints and toilets that are difficult to access).*

Transient *Temporary or occasional incontinence that may be related to a variety of causes, for example: delirium, infection, atrophic urethritis or vaginitis, some pharmaceuticals (such as sedatives/ hypnotics, diuretics, anticholinergic agents), increased urine production, restricted mobility or fecal impaction. The incontinence is transient because it is related to a potentially improvable or reversible cause.*

4. Surveyor Guidance for Incontinence Management

The following are key points from the CMS clinical guidance to surveyors for management of incontinence.

A resident should be evaluated on admission and whenever there is a change in cognition, physical ability, or urinary tract function. The type of the incontinence is a key aspect of assessment and helps identify the appropriate program/interventions to address incontinence. Use a twenty-four hour incontinence diary to record and evaluate specific information, such as, frequency and times of incontinence and toileting and response to specific interventions).

Options for managing urinary incontinence in nursing home residents include primarily behavioral programs and medication therapy:

- Bladder Rehabilitation/Bladder Retraining
- Prompted Voiding
- Habit Training/Scheduled Voiding
- Medication Therapy
- Absorbent Products

"Bladder Rehabilitation/Bladder Retraining" is a behavioral technique that requires the resident to resist or inhibit the sensation of urgency (the strong desire to urinate), to postpone or delay voiding, and to urinate according to a timetable rather than to the urge to void. Residents who are assessed with urge or mixed incontinence and are cognitively intact may be candidates for bladder retraining;

"Prompted Voiding" has three components: regular monitoring with encouragement to report continence status; prompting to toilet on a scheduled basis; and praise and positive feedback when the resident is continent and attempts to toilet. Prompted voiding focuses on teaching the resident, who is incontinent, to recognize bladder fullness or the need to void, to ask for help, or to respond when prompted to toilet. Residents who are assessed with urge or mixed incontinence and are cognitively impaired may be candidates for prompted voiding.

"Habit Training/Scheduled Voiding." Habit training includes timed voiding with the interval based on the resident's usual voiding schedule or pattern. Scheduled voiding is timed voiding, usually every three to four hours while awake. Residents who cannot self-toilet may be candidates for habit training or scheduled voiding programs.

"Medication Therapy" is used to treat specific types of incontinence, including stress incontinence and those categories associated with an overactive bladder, which may involve symptoms including urge incontinence, urinary urgency, frequency and nocturia. It is important to weigh the risks and benefits before prescribing medications for continence management and to monitor for both effectiveness and side effects.

"Absorbent Products" should not be used as the primary long term approach to continence management until the resident has been appropriately evaluated and other alternative approaches have been considered. The potential disadvantages of absorbent products are the impact on the resident's dignity, cost, the association with skin breakdown and irritation, and the amount of time needed to check and change them.

The type of incontinence management may be influenced by factors such as **resident choice** and/or **advanced directives.**

"Resident Choice." In order for a resident to exercise his or her right appropriately to make informed choices about care and treatment or to refuse treatment, the facility and the resident (or the resident's legal representative) must discuss the resident's condition, treatment options, expected outcomes, and consequences of refusing treatment. The facility should address the resident's concerns and offer relevant alternatives, if the resident has refused specific treatments.

"Advance Directives." If the facility has implemented individualized approaches for end-of-life care in accordance with the resident's wishes, and has implemented appropriate efforts to try to stabilize the resident's condition (or indicated why the condition cannot or should not be stabilized), and has provided care based on the assessed needs of the resident, then the development, continuation, or progression of urinary incontinence; the insertion and prolonged use of an indwelling urinary catheter; the development of infection or skin-related complications from urine or an indwelling catheter may be consistent with regulatory requirement.

5. Survey Procedures for Incontinence Management

Surveyors will <u>observe</u>:

- *How staff respond to the incontinence episodes; and*
- *Whether care is provided in accord with standards of practice (including infection control practices) and with*

respect for the resident's dignity.

- *Whether the resident is on a scheduled check and change program; and whether staff check and change in a timely fashion.*

- *The condition of the pads/sheets/clothing (a delay in providing continence care may be indicated by brown rings/circles, saturated linens/clothing, odors, etc.);*

- *The resident's physical condition (such as skin integrity, maceration, erythema, erosion);*

- *The resident's psychosocial outcomes (such as embarrassment or expressions of humiliation, resignation, about being incontinent);*

- *Whether staff implemented appropriate hygiene measures (e.g., cleansing, rinsing, drying and applying protective moisture barriers or barrier films as indicated) to try to prevent skin breakdown from prolonged exposure of the skin to urine.*

Surveyors will <u>interview the resident, family or responsible party</u> to identify:

- *Their involvement in care plan development including defining the approaches and goals, and whether interventions reflect preferences and choices;*

- *Their awareness of the existing continence program and how to use devices or equipment;*

- *If timely assistance is provided as needed for toileting needs, hydration and personal hygiene and if continence care and/or catheter care is provided according to the care plan;*

- *If the resident comprehends and applies information and instructions to help improve or maintain continence (where cognition permits);*

- *Presence of urinary tract-related pain, including causes and management;*

- *If interventions were refused, whether consequences and/or other alternative approaches were presented and discussed; and*

  Awareness of any current UTI, history of UTIs, or perineal skin problems.

Surveyors may interview the nursing assistants to determine if they:

- *Are aware of, and understand, the interventions specific to a particular resident (such as the bladder or bowel restorative/management programs);*

- *Know what, when, and to whom to report changes in status regarding bowel and bladder function, hydration status, urine characteristics, and complaints of urinary-related symptoms.*

Surveyors may interview the nurse responsible for coordinating or overseeing the resident's care to determine:

- *How the staff monitor implementation of the care plan, changes in continence, skin condition, and the status of UTIs;*

- *If the resident resists toileting, how staff have been taught to respond;*

- *Types of interventions that have been attempted to*

promote continence (i.e., special clothing, devices, types and frequency of assistance, change in toileting schedule, environmental modifications);

- *If the resident is not on a restorative program, how it was determined that the resident could not benefit from interventions such as a scheduled toileting program;*

- *For the resident on a program of toileting, whether the nursing staff can identify the programming applicable to the resident, and:*

    - *The type of incontinence;*

    - *The interventions to address that specific type.*

- *How it is determined that the schedule and program is effective (i.e., how continence is maintained or if there has been a decline or improvement in continence, how the program is revised to address the changes); and*

- *Whether the resident has any physical or cognitive limitations that influence potential improvement of his/her continence.*

6. Documentation Guidelines for Urinary Incontinence

IDT Team: Nurse, physician

Orders: Diagnostic tests
Medications to treat incontinence
Special appliances

Assessment: Patterns of incontinent episodes, daily voiding patterns or prior routines

Fluid intake and hydration status

Risks or conditions that may affect urinary continence

Use of medications that may affect continence and impaired continence that could reflect adverse drug reactions

Type of incontinence (stress, urge, overflow, mixed, functional, or transient incontinence) and contributing factors

Environmental factors that might facilitate or impede the ability to maintain bladder continence, such as access to the toilet, call bell, type of clothing and/or continence products, ambulation devices (walkers, canes), use of restraints, side rails

Voiding records to detect urinary patterns or intervals between incontinence episodes and facilitate planning care to avoid or reduce the frequency of episodes

Care Plan: Steps to identify cause of incontinence and treating underlying conditions

Specific type of retraining/habit/scheduled toileting program and schedule (e.g., toilet within an hour prior to each meal and within 30 minutes after meals, or check for episodes of incontinence within 30 minutes after each meal or specific times based upon the assessment of voiding patterns)

Sufficient fluid intake, including alternatives such as food substitutes that have a high liquid content, if there is reduced fluid intake

Bowel management program to meet the assessed needs

Interventions to prevent skin breakdown from prolonged exposure to urine and stool

Potential impact on continence of medication and urinary tract stimulants or irritants (e.g., caffeine) in foods and beverages; adjusting medications affecting continence (e.g., medication cessation, dose reduction, selection of an alternate medication, change in time of administration)

Managing pain for residents suffering from arthritis, contractures, neurological impairments, etc.

Environmental accommodations:

- devices such as urinals, bedpans and commodes
- handicapped toilet, elevated toilet seats, grab bars
- reducing the distance to the toilet, maintaining a clear pathway and ready access to toilet facilities
- improved lighting
- placing the call bell within reach and responding to the call bell, in relation to meeting toileting needs

Assistance to prevent incontinence episodes, such as whether prompting, transfer, and/or stand-by assist to ambulate, use of devices such as urinals

Specific frequency for a check and change program, use of pads and appliances

Progress Notes:

Ability to use the toilet, assistance with clothing, reminding resident, physical difficulties, i.e., arthritis, confusion.

Regularity, interventions for constipation diarrhea

Frequency of incontinence, frequency of changes.

Assessment of progress or regress with retraining efforts

Adequacy of fluid intake, how much and how often fluids are taken.

The frequency of breakthrough or transient incontinence;

Resident failure to comply with a continence program and alternative approaches that were offered to try to maintain or improve continence, including counseling regarding the potential consequences of not following the program

7. Surveyor Guidance for Indwelling Catheters

The following are key points from the CMS clinical guidance to surveyors for indwelling catheters.

Documentation in the clinical record must include appropriate indications for continuing use of an indwelling catheter beyond 14 days may include:

- Urinary retention that cannot be treated or corrected medically or surgically, for which alternative therapy is not feasible, and which is characterized by:

  - Documented post void residual (PVR) volumes in a range over 200 milliliters (ml);

  - Inability to manage the retention/incontinence with intermittent catheterization; and

  - Persistent overflow incontinence, symptomatic infections, and/or renal dysfunction.

- Contamination of Stage III or IV pressure ulcers with urine which has impeded healing, despite appropriate personal care for the incontinence; and

- Terminal illness or severe impairment, which makes positioning or clothing changes uncomfortable, or which is associated with intractable pain.

8. Survey Procedures for Indwelling Catheters

Surveyors will observe

- *How staff manage and assess urinary leakage from the point of catheter insertion to the bag, if present;*

- *If the resident has catheter-related pain, how staff assess and manage the pain; and*

- *What interventions (such as anchoring the catheter, avoiding excessive tugging on the catheter during transfer and care delivery) are being used to prevent inadvertent catheter removal or tissue injury from dislodging the catheter.*

- *For a resident experiencing incontinence and who has an indwelling or intermittent catheter, observe whether the resident is provided and encouraged to take enough fluids to meet the resident's hydration needs, as reflected in various measures of hydration status (approximately 30ml/kg/day or as indicated based on the resident's clinical condition).*

Surveyors will interview to determine if nursing staff

- *Can provide appropriate justification for the use of the catheter;*
- *Can identify previous attempts made (and the results of the attempts) to remove a catheter; and*
- *Can identify a history of UTIs (if present), and interventions to try to prevent recurrence.*

9. Documentation Guidelines for Indwelling Catheters

IDT Input: Nursing, physician, infection control

Assessment: The medical justification for

- for the initiation and continuing need (longer than 14 days) for catheter use,
- consideration of the risks and benefits of an indwelling (suprapubic or urethral) catheter;
- potential for removal of the catheter;
- complications resulting from the use of an indwelling catheter, such as symptoms of blockage of the catheter with associated bypassing of urine, expulsion of the catheter, pain, discomfort and bleeding.

Orders: Diagnostic tests, UA, Cultures and sensitivity
Intake and output monitoring
Type and size of catheter
Orders for catheter care, flushing, changing of catheter

Type of irrigation, the solution and any medications to be used and frequency

Care Plan: Defines the type of catheter, tubing and bag care, including indications, according to facility protocol, for changing the catheter, tubing or bag

Minimize catheter-related injury, pain, encrustation, excessive urethral tension, accidental removal, or obstruction of urine outflow

Keeping the catheter anchored to prevent excessive tension on the catheter, which can lead to urethral tears or dislodging the catheter; and securing the catheter to facilitate flow of urine

Minimize risk of infection (personal hygiene measures such as handwashing and catheter/tubing/bag care)

Sufficient fluid intake, including alternatives such as food substitutes that have a high liquid content, if there is reduced fluid intake

Assess potential evidence of symptomatic UTI or other related changes in urine condition (such as onset of bloody urine, cloudiness, or oliguria, if present)

Assessment and removal of the indwelling catheter when no longer needed

Monitoring for excessive post void residual, after removing a catheter that was inserted for obstruction or overflow incontinence

Notify the physician of the resident's condition

or changes in the resident's continence status or development of symptoms that may represent a symptomatic UTI (in contrast to asymptomatic bacteriuria

Progress Notes:

Special needs for foley catheter flow and verification the catheter is patent

Color, consistency, odor and quality of urine

Resident tolerance to irrigations

Indications for catheter changes, any problems or difficulties in insertion

Assessment for symptoms of UTI and abdominal distension, notification of physician if symptoms develop

Observe for complications resulting from the continuing use of the catheter, such as obstruction resulting from catheter encrustation, urethral erosion, bladder spasms, hematuria, and leakage around the catheter

Adequacy of fluid intake, how much fluid offered and how often

10. Surveyor guidance for UTI

The following are key points from the CMS clinical guidance for prevention of urinary tract infection.

Urinary tract infection (UTI) is one of the most common infections occurring in nursing homes and is often related to an indwelling urinary catheter. Without a valid clinical rationale for an indwelling catheter, its use is not an acceptable approach to manage urinary incontinence. Although UTIs can result from the resident's own flora, they may also be the result of microorganisms transmitted by staff when handling the urinary catheter drainage system and/or providing incontinence care. Hand washing remains one of the most effective infection control tools available.

Because many residents have chronic bacteriuria, the research-based literature suggests treating only symptomatic UTIs. Symptomatic UTIs are based on the following criteria:

- Residents without a catheter should have at least three of the following signs and symptoms:
    - Fever (increase in temperature of >2 degrees F (1.1 degrees C) or rectal temperature >99.5 degrees F (37.5 degrees C) or single measurement of temperature >100 degrees F (37.8 degrees C));
    - New or increased burning pain on urination, frequency or urgency;
    - New flank or suprapubic pain or tenderness;
    - Change in character of urine (e.g., new bloody urine, foul smell, or amount of sediment) or as reported by the laboratory (new pyuria or microscopic hematuria); and/or
    - Worsening of mental or functional status (e.g., confusion, decreased appetite, unexplained falls, incontinence of recent onset, lethargy, decreased activity).

- Residents <u>with a catheter</u> should have at least two of the following signs and symptoms:

    - Fever or chills;

    - New flank pain or suprapubic pain or tenderness;

    - Change in character of urine (e.g., new bloody urine, foul smell, or amount of sediment) or as reported by the laboratory (new pyuria or microscopic hematuria); and/or

    - Worsening of mental or functional status. Local findings such as obstruction, leakage, or mucosal trauma (hematuria) may also be present.

11. Survey Procedures for UTI

Surveyors will <u>observe:</u>

- *Determine if staff wash their hands after providing incontinence care, and before and after providing catheter care.*

Surveyors will <u>interview family</u>

- *Awareness of any current UTI, history of UTIs, or perineal skin problems.*

12. Documentation Guidelines for UTI

<u>IDT input:</u> Nursing, infection control, physician

<u>Assessment:</u> Fluid needs and implement a fluid management program (using alternative approaches as needed) based on those assessed needs

Recurrent UTIs (2 or more in 6 months). Factors possibly contributing to chronically recurring or persistent UTIs

In a noncatheterized resident

- rule out structural abnormalities such as enlarged prostate, prolapsed bladder, periurethral abscess, strictures, bladder calculi, polyps and tumors (such as a determination of an abnormal post void residual (PVR) urine volume or a referral to a urologist)
- check perineal hygiene performed in accordance with accepted practices

In a catheterized resident

- possible impairment of free urine flow through the catheter
- re-evaluate the techniques being used for perineal hygiene and catheter care, and
- reconsider the relative risks and benefits of continuing the use of an indwelling catheter

Order: Diagnostic Tests
Medications
Hydration
Monitoring of vital signs

Care Plan: Medication and treatment ordered
Fluid intake, how much and how often fluids are to be offered
Monitoring of vital signs
Infection control procedures in managing catheters and associated drainage system

Progress Notes:

Medications and treatment ordered, response to medications, observation of side effects

Adequacy of fluids taken, how much and how often consumed

Monitoring of vital signs, assessment of signs and symptoms of infection

Infection control procedures implemented

Temporary restrictions on activities

RANGE OF MOTION

Range of motion means the extent of movement of a joint. Decline in the residents ability to move may be due to immobility, stroke, injury or surgical procedure.

Preventative care is provided to prevent further limitation of movement or muscle atrophy. Active ROM may be performed by the resident; passive ROM performed by staff or active-assistive ROM exercises may be performed by the resident and the staff. It may be necessary to apply splints or braces.

1. Federal Regulations

Federal regulations for quality of care section 483.25(e) address the prevention of decrease in range of motion.

***(e)* Range of Motion.**

Based on the comprehensive assessment of a resident, the facility must ensure that--

(1) A resident who enters the facility without a limited range of motion does not experience reduction in range of motion unless the resident's clinical condition demonstrates that a reduction in range of motion is unavoidable; and

(2) A resident with a limited range of motion

> ***receives appropriate treatment and services to increase range of motion and/or to prevent further decrease in range of motion.***

The intent of this regulation is to ensure that the resident reaches and maintains his or her highest level of range of motion and to prevent avoidable decline of range of motion.

2. Quality Measures/Indicators

The following quality measures/indicators are calculated on data submitted on the MDS surveyors will review these measures before visiting the facility to identify focus areas for review.

9.4 Incidence in decline in ROM

3. Surveyor Guidance

The surveyor guidelines state that a resident will receive adequate preventative care to avoid development or increase of contractures. Clinical conditions that are *primary risk factors* for a decreased range of motion are:

- Immobilization (e.g., bedfast)
- Deformities arising out of neurological deficits (e.g., strokes, multiple sclerosis, cerebral palsy, and polio)
- Pain, spasms, and immobility associated with arthritis or late stage Alzheimer's disease

Reduction in ROM may be unavoidable if limbs or digits are immobilized because of injury or surgical procedure.

4. Survey Procedures

The surveyor procedures instruct the surveyor to sample resident charts for residents who need routine care to prevent contractures.

- *For residents who have limited ROM, what is the facility doing to prevent further declines in ROM?*

- *Are passive ROM exercises provided and active ROM exercises supervised per the plan of care?*

- *Have care plan objectives and resident progress been evaluated?*

- *Is there evidence that care planning is changed as the resident's condition changes?*

- *Identify if resident triggers RAPS for ADL functional/rehabilitation potential, visual function, and communication. Consider whether the RAPs used to assess causal factors for decline, potential for decline or lack of improvement.*

- *Is there evidence that there has been a decline in residents' ROM or muscle atrophy that was avoidable?*

- *Was the resident at risk for decline in ROM? If so, why?*

- *What care did the facility provide, including routine preventive measures that addressed the resident's unique risk factors (e.g., use muscle strengthening exercises in residents with muscle atrophy)?*

- *Was this care provided consistently?*

- *Reduction of ROM is unavoidable only if adequate*

assessment, appropriate care planning, and preventive care was provided and resulted in limitation in ROM or muscle atrophy.

5. Documentation Guidelines for Range of Motion

IDT Input: Nursing, restorative therapy, activity, social services

Orders:

Referral to physical therapist
Special appliances and devices
Limitations on weight bearing and/or activity, requirement for bed rest

Plan:

Active passive exercises, frequency
Positioning frequency and type for correct body alignment
Special appliances and devices
Evaluation by physical therapy
Activity exercise programs

Progress Notes:

Ability of resident to move joints without pain.
Any reduction or increase of ability to move joints.
Frequency and response to ROM and activity exercise programs
Response to any appliances or devices used to prevent further contractures.
Describe clinical conditions that are primary risk for decreased range of motion.
Deformities arising out of neurological deficits (e.g. strokes, multiple sclerosis, cerebral palsy and polio)
Pain, spasms, and immobility associated with arthritis or late stages of Alzheimer's disease

MENTAL AND PSYCHOSOCIAL FUNCTIONING

Dementia and behavioral problems often go hand in hand for nursing home residents. Residents in nursing homes who are already coping with the loss of mental ability can become overwhelmed by a sense of loss of their capabilities, of family and friends, of their possessions, and of the ability to continue to pursue activities and hobbies.

Mental and psychosocial adjustment refers to problems residents have in adapting to changes in life's circumstances. In the MDS/RAI process, there are five (5) Resident Assessment Protocols that address these needs:

Delirium
Cognitive Loss/Dementia
Psychosocial Well-being
Mood State
Behavioral Symptoms

1. Federal Regulations

Section 483.25(f) addresses the management of mental and psychosocial adjustment difficulties.

(f) ***Mental and Psychosocial functioning.***

Based on the comprehensive assessment of a resident, the

facility must ensure that--

(1) ***A resident who displays mental or psychosocial adjustment difficulty, receives appropriate treatment and services to correct the assessed problems, and***

(2) ***A resident whose assessment did not reveal a mental or psychosocial adjustment difficulty does not display a pattern of decreased social interaction and/or increase in withdrawn, angry, or depressive behaviors, unless the resident's clinical condition demonstrates that such a pattern was unavoidable.***

The intent of this regulation is that the resident receives care and services to assist him or her to reach and maintain the highest level of mental and psychosocial functioning.

2. Quality Measures/Indicators

The following quality measures/indicators are calculated on data submitted on the MDS. Surveyors will review these measures before visiting the facility to identify focus areas for review.

2.1 Residents who have become more depressed or anxious

2.2 Prevalence of behavior symptoms affecting others

2.3 Prevalence of symptoms of depression without antidepressant therapy

4.1 Incidence of cognitive impairment

3. Surveyor Guidance

The surveyor guidance states that manifestations of mental and psychosocial adjustment difficulties may, over a period of time, include:

- Impaired verbal communication,
- Social isolation (e.g., loss or failure to have relationships),
- Sleep pattern disturbance (e.g., disruptive change in sleep or rest pattern as related to one's biological and emotional needs),
- Spiritual distress (disturbances in one's belief system),
- Inability to control behavior and potential for violence (aggressive behavior directed at self or others.),
- Stereotyped response to any stressor (i.e., the same characteristic response, regardless of the stimulus).

Clinical conditions that may produce apathy, malaise, and decrease energy levels that can be mistaken for depression associated with mental or psychosocial adjustment difficulty are:

- Metabolic disease (e.g., abnormalities of serum glucose, potassium, calcium and blood urea nitrogen, hepatic dysfunction),
- Endocrine disease (e.g., hypothyroidism, hyperthyroidism, diabetes, hypoparathyroidism, hyperparathyroidism, Cushing's disease, Addison's disease),
- Central nervous system diseases (e.g., tumors and other mass lesions, Parkinson's disease, multiple sclerosis, Alzheimer's disease, vascular disease),
- Miscellaneous disease (e.g., pernicious anemia, pancreatic disease, malignancy, infections, congestive heart failure),
- Over-medication with anti-hypertensive drugs,
- Presence of restraints.

4. Survey Procedures

The survey procedures instruct the surveyor to sample

resident charts for residents exhibiting difficulties in mental and psychosocial adjustment.

- *Is there a complete accurate assessment of resident's usual and customary routines?*

- *What evidence is there that the facility makes accommodations for the resident's usual and customary routines?*

- *What programs/activities has the resident received to improve and maintain maximum mental and psychosocial functioning?*

- *Has the resident's mental and psychosocial functioning been maintained or improved (e.g., fewer symptoms of distress)? Have treatment plans and objectives been re-evaluated?*

- *Has the resident received a psychological or psychiatric evaluation to evaluate, diagnose, or treat her/his condition, if necessary?*

- *Identify if resident triggers RAPS for activities, mood state, psychosocial well-being, and psychotropic drug use. Consider whether the RAPs were used to assess the causal factors for decline, potential for decline or lack of improvement.*

- *How are mental and psychosocial adjustment difficulties addressed in the care plan?*

For residents whose assessment did not reveal a mental or psychosocial adjustment difficulty, but who display decreased social interaction or increased withdrawn, angry, or depressed behaviors, determine if this behavior was unavoidable.

- *Did the facility attempt to evaluate whether this behavior was attributable to organic causes or other risk factors not associated with adjusting to living in the nursing facility?*

- *What care did the resident receive to maintain his/her mental or psychosocial functioning?*

- *Were individual objectives of the plan of care periodically evaluated, and if progress was not made in reducing, maintaining, or increasing behaviors that assist the resident to have his/her needs meet, were alternative treatment approaches developed to maintain mental or psychosocial functioning?*

- *Identify if resident triggers RAPs for behavioral symptoms, cognitive loss/dementia, and psychosocial well-being. Consider whether the RAPs were used to assess causal factors for decline, potential for decline or lack of improvement.*

- *Did the facility use the RAPs for behavioral symptoms, cognitive loss/dementia and psychosocial well-being to assess why the behaviors or change is mental or psychosocial functioning was occurring?*

5. Documentation Guidelines for Delirium

IDT Team: Nursing, social services, activity, pharmacist, psychologist, psychiatrist, physician

Orders: Review of resident's drug profile by a physician
Consultation from psychologist or psychiatrist
Diagnostic tests
Orders for treatment of underlying cause of delirium

Care Plan: Observe for acute, reversible causes of delirium
Treatment of underlying cause of delirium
Environment conducive to reducing symptoms
Interventions to maintain resident's customary routines and adjustment to facility
Task segmentation/ADL support
Emotional support, reassurance

Progress Notes:

Description of signs and symptoms of delirium

Observations of situations when signs and symptoms occur. Coping ability of resident with change in functional level

Response to treatment for underlying cause of delirium

Response to reality orientation, activity programs, psychosocial support and interventions

6. Documentation Guidelines for Cognitive Loss/Dementia

IDT Input: Nursing, social services, activity

Orders: Review resident's drug profile with a physician
Diagnostic tests

Care Plan: Develop care plans focused on three main goals

- to provide positive experiences for the resident (e.g., enjoyable activities) that do not involve overly demanding tasks and stress;
- to define appropriate support roles for staff involved in residents' care;

- to lay the foundation for reasonable staff and family expectations concerning a resident's capacities and needs.

Participation in appropriate diversional activity programs

- Reality orientation, Task segmentation/ and.or Validation
- Family/Peer/Volunteer support

Accommodation of customary routines, if resident's condition allows

Management of sleep disturbance and cognitive deficit related problem behavior

Interventions to reduce sensory dysfunction and optimize orientation, hearing, vision and communication deficits

Progress Notes:

Ability to remember short and long term events.

Response to task segmentation or cuing for task performance.

Response to social interactions and involvement in daily life at the facility.

Extent of family involvement

Response to activity programs

Behavior management programs, identification of stressors

Ability to see, hear and communicate effectively with staff and family

7. Documentation Guidelines for Psychosocial Well-being

IDT Team: Nursing, social services, activity, psychologist, psychiatrist

Care Plan: Systematic orientation programs

Involvement in facility daily life, activity programs, goal setting, providing residents with opportunities for self-governance

Development of positive relationships with staff, other residents, family and volunteers

Arrangements to keep resident in touch with their communities, cultural heritage, former lifestyle and religious practices.

Referral to social worker or psychologist

Progress Notes:

Treatment and services offered for self-governance and response to opportunities for choices

Contacts with social and community groups

Involvement with facility activity program

Extent of family or significant others involvement in care

8. Documentation Guidelines for Mood State

IDT Team: Nursing, social services, activity, psychologist, psychiatrist

Orders: Review of resident drug regime with physician
Referrals for consultant by psychologist, psychiatrist
Diagnostic tests

Care Plan: Steps to identify confounding problems, signs and symptoms of depression
Environmental changes and adaptations
Resident strengths and resources
Family/volunteer involvement
Referral to social worker or psychologist
Participation in activity programs
Antidepressant therapy

Prevention of mood decline

- Orientation of new residents
- Assist resident to be as independent as possible
- Pursuit of meaningful activities
- Making connections with the past
- Grief interventions

Progress Notes:

Description of manifestation of mood disturbance, circumstances when mood variations occur.
Response to opportunities for self-governance
Effectiveness of systematic orientation program
Contacts with social and community groups, involvement with facility activity program

Response to antidepressant therapy and observations for side effects of drugs

9. Documentation Guidelines for Behavioral Symptoms

IDT Team: Nursing, social service, activity, psychologist, psychiatrist

Orders: Review of resident drug regime with physician
Referrals for consultant by psychologist, psychiatrist
Diagnostic tests

Care Plan: Involvement in appropriate activity programs
Behavioral management program,
Crisis intervention services, if warranted.
Observation for underlying cause of behavior/ non-drug interventions.
Psychotropic drug therapy and monitoring.
Changes in environmental conditions, identification of stressors
Referral to social worker or psychologist

Progress Notes:

Observations for mental dysfunctions such as sad or anxious mood

Motivation toward health care

Descriptions of behaviors:

- yelling, screaming or moaning
- fighting, cursing, arguing
- wandering, unsafe movement
- resisting care
- sleep problems

- anxiety, fearfulness
- inappropriate sexual behavior
- delusions, hallucinations

Interactions with family, activities, staff, other residents

Adjustment to the facility and to physical and mental limitations.

Involvement in life around them, sense of dissatisfaction with life, meaningful activity pursuits

<u>Behavior management program</u>

- Immediate action to bring dangerous or disruptive behavior under control
- Medical evaluation for physical causes, social psychological or environmental causes
- Behavior assessment to identify the behavior of most concern
- Use behavior assessment log to record how often behavior occurs
- Gather information on possible causes of behavior
- Observe responses to staff interventions

FEEDING TUBES

Decisions about the appropriateness of tube feeding for a resident are developed with the resident or his/her family, surrogate or representative as part of determining the care plan.

Residents who are being fed by naso-gastric tubes often qualify for Medicare Part A reimbursement. To demonstrate skilled nursing, daily charting must be recorded by the licensed nurse. Narrative notes are written to evaluate the maintenance of nutrition and monitor for complications. Staff needs to be constantly alert to the incidence of complications from feeding tubes. Complications in tube feeding are not necessarily the result of improper care.

Flow sheets may also be used in addition to the narrative charting to document and compare the skilled care being provided. The flow sheet can be used to record feedings given, maintenance of the tube and tube site, checking for residuals, as well as observations for complications and positioning of the resident.

1. Federal Regulations

Section 483.25(g) addresses the care of residents who require tube feeding.

(g) ***<u>Naso-gastric tubes</u>***

Based on the comprehensive assessment of a resident, the

facility must ensure that--

(1) A resident who has been able to eat enough alone or with assistance is not fed by naso-gastric tube unless the resident's clinical condition demonstrates that use of a naso-gastric tube was unavoidable; and

(2) A resident who is fed by a naso-gastric or gastrostomy tube receives the appropriate treatment and services to prevent aspiration pneumonia, diarrhea, vomiting, dehydration, metabolic abnormalities, and nasal-pharyngeal ulcers and to restore, if possible, normal feeding function.

The intent of this regulation is that a naso-gastric tube feeding is utilized only after adequate assessment, and the resident's clinical condition makes this treatment necessary. This requirement is also intended to prevent the use of tube feeding when ordered over the objection of the resident. As part of the admission process identification of any advance directives made by the resident prior to admission should be documented in the clinical record.

2. Quality Measures/Indicators

The following quality measures/indicators are calculated on data submitted on the MDS. Surveyors will review these measures before visiting the facility to identify focus areas for review.

7.2 Prevalence of Tube Feeding

3. Surveyor Guidance

Surveyors are asked to evaluate residents who are receiving nourishments via feeding tubes. The record must contain justification of the need for the use of the feeding tube.

Clinical conditions demonstrating that nourishment via a naso-gastric tube is unavoidable include:

- The inability to swallow without choking or aspiration such as in cases of Parkinson's disease, pseudobulbar palsy, or esophageal diverticulum,

- Lack of sufficient alertness for oral nutrition (e.g., resident comatose),

- Malnutrition not attributable to a single cause or causes that can be isolated and reversed. There is documented evidence that the facility has not been able to maintain or improve the resident's nutritional status through oral intake.

4. Survey Procedures

For residents who, upon admission to the facility, were not tube fed and now have a feeding tube, determine if tube feeding was unavoidable.

- *Did the facility identify the resident for malnutrition?*

- *What did the facility do to maintain oral feeding, prior to inserting a feeding tube? Did staff provide assistance in eating? Did staff cue resident as needed, assist with the use of assistive devices, or feed the resident, if necessary?*

- *Is the resident receiving therapy to improve or enhance swallowing skills?*

- *Was an assessment done to determine the cause of deceased oral intake/weight loss or malnutrition?*

- *If there was a dietitian consultation, were recommendations followed?*

For all sampled residents <u>who are tube fed</u>:

- *Is the NG tube properly placed?*

- *Are staff responsibilities for providing enteral feedings clearly assigned (i.e., who administers the feeding, formula, amount, feeding intervals, flow rate)?*

- *Do staff monitor feeding complications (e.g., diarrhea, gastric distension, aspiration) and administer corrective actions to allay complications (e.g., changing rate of formula administration)?*

- *Are there negative consequences of tube use (e.g., agitation, depression, self-extubation, infections, aspiration and restraint use without a medical reason for the restraint)?*

- *When long term use is anticipated, is G tube placement considered?*

Is the potential for <u>complications from feeding</u> minimized by:

- *Use of a small bore, flexible naso-gastric tube, unless contraindicated.*

- *Securely attaching the tube to the nose/face.*

- *Checking for correct tube placement prior to beginning a feeding or administering medications and after episodes of vomiting or suctioning.*

- *Checking a resident with a newly inserted gastric tube for gastric residual volume every 2-4 hours until the resident has demonstrated an ability to empty his/her stomach*

- *Properly elevating the resident's head*

- *Providing the type, rate and volume of the feeding as ordered*

- *Using universal precautions and clean technique and as per facility/manufacturer's directions when stopping, starting, flushing, and giving medications through the tube;*

- *Using hang time recommendations by the manufacturer to prevent excessive microbial growth;*

- *Implement the procedures to ensure cleanliness of supplies, e.g. irrigating syringes changed on a regular bases as per facility policy. It is not necessary to change the irrigating syringe each time it is used;*

- *Using a pump equipped with a functional alarm (if pump used)*

- *The facility's criteria for determining that a resident may be able to return to eating by mouth (e.g., a resident whose Parkinson's symptoms have been controlled)*
  - -- *If so, the facility has assisted them in returning to normal eating.*

- *Identify if resident triggers RAPs for feeding tubes, nutritional status, and dehydration/fluid maintenance. Consider whether the RAPs were used to assess causal factors for decline, potential for decline and lack of improvement.*

5. Documentation Guidelines for Feeding Tubes

IDT Team: Nursing, dietary, social service, speech therapy, occupational therapy

Assessment: Diagnosis justifying use.

Orders:
Formula, type, rate of feeding, calories, additional water
Type of tube used
Schedule for flushing tube
Supplemental nourishments
Weaning off tube
Intake and Output/Monitoring of weights
Occupational or speech therapy
Advance Directives

Care Plan:
Type of tube, insertion type, rate and volume of feeding
Checking tube for placement
Use of pump/Aseptic technique
Positioning of resident, elevation of head
Interventions to prevent complications
Observation for complications
Intake and output
Target body weight, frequency of monitoring weights
Occupational or speech therapy program
Advance directives

Progress Notes:

Enteral Flow sheet:
- Formula, Calories/24 hrs, CC/Hr
- Via pump/gravity
- Flush with ___cc water/frequency
- Formula bag + tubing checked to assure

they have been changed within last 36 hours

- Tube site care once per day
- Change syringe q day, label with date.
- Head elevation
- Verify tube placement
- Oral care
- Check for residual q shift

Check for complications:

- formula intolerance,
- breath sounds,
- signs of dehydration

Narrative Assessment:

- Assess response and toleration of feeding
- Problems with tube placement
  removal and reinsertion
  signs and symptoms of aspiration
- Observations of bowel problems, adequate hydration,
  skin and mouth problems.
- Physical limitations or resident response to tube feeding
- Other sources of nutrition, if any
- Weight fluctuations

ACCIDENT HAZARDS AND PREVENTION

An **"accident"** is an unexpected, unintended event that can cause a resident bodily injury. Identification of accident hazards and which residents are at risk for falls is necessary to maintain a safe environment. On admission all residents should be assessed for falls risk. Immediate precautions could include orientation to the facility and increased monitoring while the resident adjusts to the new environment.

The comprehensive MDS triggers falls risk annually and when there is a significant change of condition. Residents with poor balance or who use psychotherapeutic drugs have a high risk for an initial fall. Other risk factors, such as, cardiovascular disease, neuromuscular dysfunction, orthopedic problems, impaired hearing and sensory perception can contribute to the potential risk for falls. Those at risk for falls should have care plan interventions to prevent, if possible, further falls.

Residents who have fallen once have a high risk to fall again. An aggressive program for falls prevention evaluates every fall for causative factors. Consideration should be given to environmental factors, wheelchair and seating arrangements, use of psychotropic drugs and transferring and ambulation.

After each fall, the facility is expected to analyze the causal factors that may have contributed. The care plan interventions are updated based on a post fall assessment. Staff implements these new interventions to prevent similar accidents or falls.

1. Federal Regulations

Section 483.25(h) addresses the prevention of accidents and accident hazards.

(h) ***Accidents***

The facility must ensure that--

(1) The resident environment remains as free of accident hazards as is possible; and

(2) Each resident receives adequate supervision and assistance devices to prevent accidents.

The intent of this provision is that the facility prevents accidents by providing an environment that is as free from hazards over which the facility has control. The facility will identify each resident at risk for accidents and/or falls, and adequately plan care and implement procedures to prevent accidents.

2. Quality Measures/Indicators

The following quality measures/indicators are calculated on data submitted on the MDS. Surveyors will review these measures before visiting the facility to identify focus areas for review.

1.1 Incidence of new fractures

1.2 Prevalence of falls

3. Definitions

The surveyor guidance provides the following definitions:

Accident *An unexpected, unintended event that can cause a resident bodily injury.*

Accident hazard *Physical features in the nursing facility environment that can endanger a resident's safety, including but not limited to:*

- *Physical restraints;*
- *Equipment or devices that are defective, poorly maintained, or not used in accordance with manufacturer's specifications*
- *Bathing facilities that do not have non-slip surfaces;*
- *Hazards (e.g., electrical appliances with frayed wires, cleaning supplies easily accessible to cognitively impaired residents, wet floors that are not obviously labeled and to which access is not blocked);*
- *Defective or improperly latched side rails or spaces within side rails, between upper and lower rails, between rails and the mattress, between side rails and the bed frame, or spaces between side rails and the head or foot board of the bed that can entrap limbs, neck or thorax, and can cause injury or death;*
- *Handrails not securely fixed to the wall, difficult to grasp, and/or with sharp edges/splinters;*
- *Water temperatures in hand sinks or bath tubs which can scald or harm residents.*

4. Survey Procedures

If a resident has had an accident, the surveyor is instructed to review the facility's investigation of that accident and their response to prevent the accident from recurring.

- *Identify if resident triggers RAPs for falls, cognitive loss/ dementia, physical restraints, and psychotropic drugs and whether the RAPs were used to assess causal factors for decline or lack of improvement.*

- *If the survey team identifies a number of or pattern of accidents, review the quality assurance activities of the facility to determine the facility's response to accidents.*
  - -- *Are there a number of accidents or injuries of a specific type or on any specific shift (e.g., falls, skin injuries)?*
  - -- *Are residents who smoke properly supervised and monitored?*

- *If the survey team identifies residents repeatedly involved in accidents or sampled residents who have had an accident:*
  - -- *Is the resident assessed for being at risk for falls?*
  - -- *What care-planning and implementation is the facility doing to prevent accidents and falls for those residents identified at risk?*
  - -- *How did the facility fit, and monitor, the use of that resident's assistive devices?*
  - -- *How were drugs that may cause postural hypotension, dizziness, or visual changes monitored?*

5. Documentation Guidelines for Falls

IDT Team: Nursing, restorative therapy

Assessment: Admission falls risk screening
Update falls risk quarterly

Orders: Orders for safety devices
Restorative evaluations and programs for strengthening
Review of medication regime with physician

Care Plan: Identification of residents at risk for falls
Use of safety devices/evaluation of seating arrangements or wheelchairs
Physical therapy programs for endurance
Increased supervision or observation
Monitor medications and potential for hypotension, dizziness of visual decline
Evaluate and update care plan if resident has fallen with new interventions or modification of present interventions

Progress Notes:

Observations of resident's usual pattern of interaction with his/her environment

- Ability to perform ADL function
- Distance and quality of ambulation
- Observance of high risk activities
- Proper seating arrangement or wheelchair fitting

Describe the circumstances of any fall

- Time of day, time since last meal
- Was resident doing usual or unusual activity?
- Was he/she standing still or walking? Reaching up or down? Not reaching?
- Was resident in a crowd of people?
- Responding to bladder/bowel urgency?

- Was there glare or liquid on floors? Foreign objects in walkway?
- New furniture placement or other changes in environment?

Take necessary vital signs
Observations for effects of medications such as hypotension, dizziness, visual changes
Notification of physician of falls/injury
Notification of family or responsible person

NUTRITION

The nutritional status of the resident is monitored by regularly scheduled weights. To be useful, consistent procedures must be followed when weighing residents. If necessary, reweigh the resident to verify accuracy.

Interventions are started immediately for unplanned weight loss to avoid complications of malnutrition. Residents are also observed for weight gain and peripheral edema. Weight loss or gain should be assessed taking into consideration the resident's former life style as well as current diagnosis.

Laboratory tests are useful in evaluating the resident's nutritional status. Although there is no requirement that specific tests be performed, it is suggested that laboratory tests, such as albumin, plasma transferrin, hemoglobin, hematocrit, potassium and magnesium be reviewed to evaluate a resident's nutritional status. Abnormal values will be expected in the elderly and in certain disease processes. **Lab results should be considered only in combination with the resident's total clinical picture.**

Monthly weights are reviewed to assure prompt interventions to weight changes. Gain or loss of 5% in 30 days or 10% in 180 are evaluated and reported to the physician.

1. Federal Regulations

Section 483.25(i) addresses the nutritional needs of

residents.

(i) *Nutrition:*

Based on a resident's comprehensive assessment, the facility must ensure that a resident --

(1) ***Maintains acceptable parameters of nutritional status, such as body weight and protein levels, unless the resident's clinical condition demonstrates that this is not possible; and***

(2) ***Receives a therapeutic diet when there is a nutritional problem.***

The intent of this regulation is to assure that the resident maintains acceptable parameters of nutritional status, taking into account the resident's clinical condition or other appropriate interventions, when there is a nutritional problem. Parameters of nutritional status, which are unacceptable, include unplanned weight loss as well as other indices such as peripheral edema, cachexia and laboratory tests indicating malnourishment (e.g., serum albumin levels).

2. Quality Measures/Indicators

The following quality measures/indicators are calculated on data submitted on the MDS. Surveyors will review these measures before visiting the facility to identify focus areas for review.

7.1 Residents who lose too much weight

3. Definitions

The guidance for surveyors provides the following definition for therapeutic diets.

Therapeutic Diet

A diet ordered by a physician as part of treatment for a disease or clinical condition, to eliminate or decrease certain substances in the diet, (e.g., sodium) or to increase certain substances in the diet (e.g., potassium), or to provide food the resident is able to eat (e.g., a mechanically altered diet).

4. Surveyor Guidance

Since ideal body weight charts have not yet been validated for the institutionalized elderly, weight loss (or gain) is a guide in determining nutritional status. An analysis of weight loss or gain should be examined in light of the individual's former life style, usual weight throughout adult life as well as the current diagnosis.

Suggested parameters for evaluating significance of unplanned and undesired weight loss are:

Interval	Significant Loss	Severe Loss
1 month	5%	Greater than 5%
3 months	7.5%	Greater than 7.5%
6 months	10%	Greater than 10%

Potential indicators of malnutrition are pale skin, dull eyes, swollen lips and gums, swollen and/or dry tongue with scarlet or magenta hue, poor skin turgor, cachexia, bilateral edema and muscle wasting.

Risk factors for malnutrition are:

- Drug therapy that may contribute to nutritional deficiencies such as:
  - Cardiac glycosides,
  - Diuretics,

  - -- Anti-inflammatory drugs,
  - -- Antacids (antacid overuse),
  - -- Laxatives (laxative overuse),
  - -- Psychotropic drug overuse,
  - -- Anticonvulsants,
  - -- Antineoplastic drugs,
  - -- Phenothiazines,
  - -- Oral hypoglycemics,
- Poor oral health status or hygiene, eyesight, motor coordination, or taste alterations,
- Depression or dementia,
- Therapeutic or mechanically altered diet,
- Lack of access to culturally acceptable foods,
- Slow eating pace resulting in food becoming unpalatable, or in staff removing the tray before resident has finished eating; and
- Cancer.

Clinical conditions demonstrating that the maintenance of acceptable nutritional status <u>may not</u> be possible include, but are not limited to:

- Refusal to eat and refusal of other methods of nourishment,
- Advanced disease (i.e., cancer, malabsorption syndrome),
- Increased nutritional/caloric needs associated with pressure sores and wound healing (e.g., fractures, burns),
- Radiation or chemotherapy,
- Kidney disease, alcohol/drug abuse, chronic blood loss, hyperthyroidism,
- Gastrointestinal surgery,
- Prolonged nausea, vomiting, diarrhea not relieved by treatment given according to accepted standards of practice.

5. Survey Procedures

The guidance to surveyors states that charts are to be reviewed to determine if residents have maintained acceptable parameter of nutritional status.

- *Where indicated by the resident's medical status, have clinically appropriate therapeutic diets been prescribed?*

For residents whose nutritional status is inadequate, determine if clinical conditions demonstrate that maintenance of inadequate nutritional status was unavoidable.

- *Did the facility identify factors that put the resident at risk for malnutrition?*

- *Identify if resident triggered RAPs for nutritional status, ADL functional/ rehabilitation potential, feeding tubes, psychotropic drug use, and dehydration/fluid balance. Consider whether the RAPs were used to assess the causal factors for decline, potential for decline or lack of improvement.*

- *What routine preventive measures and care did the resident receive to address unique risk factors for malnutrition (e.g., provision of an adequate diet with supplements or modifications as indicated by nutrient needs)?*

- *Were staff responsibilities for maintaining nutritional status clear, including monitoring the amount of food the resident is eating at each meal and offering substitutes?*

- *Was this care provided consistently?*

- *Were individual goals of the plan of care periodically evaluated and if not met, were alternative approaches considered or attempted?*

6. Documentation Guidelines for Nutrition

IDT Input: Nursing, dietary, occupational therapy

Assessment: Usual weight through adult life
Potential for weight loss
Need for weight management
Edema
Refusal to eat
If newly admitted and obese, are fewer calories provided than prior to admission

Orders: Type of therapeutic diet
Consistency of diet if other than regular
Supplemental nourishments

Diagnostic laboratory tests
- Albumin
- Plasma Transferrin
- Hemoglobin
- Hematocrit
- Potassium
- Magnesium

Care Plan: Type and consistency of diet
Additional or supplemental nourishments
Method of feeding and appliances used
Target body weight
Food preferences

Progress Notes:

Eating:
- Ability to feed oneself and drink fluids
- Ability to handle utensils

- Difficulty in chewing/swallowing assistance provided
- motivation in eating, need for cueing
- adequate nourishment

Supplemental nourishments, frequency and tolerance
Acceptance and compliance with therapeutic diet
Notification of physician of weight changes
Notification of family/responsible person of weight changes

For resident unable to maintain good nutrition, assistance provided such as

- hand feeding of foods,
- syringe feeding,
- tube feeding provided through naso-gastric or gastrostomy tube,
- total parenteral nutrition provided through a central intravenous line

HYDRATION

Sufficient fluid intake for nursing home residents is necessary to prevent dehydration. The problem may be compounded by the resident's difficulty in drinking fluids or acute illness, such as, fever that may have altered fluid and electrolyte balance.

Early detection of risk of dehydration must be identified to avoid possible complications and harm to the resident. Symptoms of dehydration are sometimes vague and unreliable. Conditions may include: dizziness, confusion, decreased urinary output, poor skin turgor, constipation and fever.

1. Federal Regulation

Section 483.25(j) addressed the need to maintain adequate hydration.

(j) Hydration.

The facility must provide each resident with sufficient fluid intake to maintain proper hydration and health.

The intent of this regulation is to assure that the resident receives sufficient amount of fluids based on individual needs to prevent dehydration.

2. Quality Measures/Indicators

The following quality measures/indicators are calculated on data submitted on the MDS. Surveyors will review these measures before visiting the facility to identify focus areas for review.

7.3 Prevalence of dehydration

3. Definitions

The survey guidance provides the following definition.

Sufficient fluid

The amount of fluid needed to prevent dehydration (output of fluids far exceeds fluid intake) and maintain health. The amount needed is specific for each resident, and fluctuates as the resident's condition fluctuates (e.g., increase fluids if resident has fever or diarrhea).

4. Surveyor Guidance

The surveyors clinical guidance provide the following key points. Risk factors for the resident becoming dehydrated are:

- Coma/decreased sensorium,
- Fluid loss and increased fluid needs (e.g., diarrhea, fever, uncontrolled diabetes),
- Fluid restriction secondary to renal dialysis,
- Functional impairments that make it difficult to drink, reach fluids, or communicate fluid needs (e.g., aphasia)
- Dementia in which resident forgets to drink; or forgets how to drink,
- Refusal of fluids.

A general guideline for determining baseline daily fluids needs is to multiply the resident's body weight in kg times 30cc (2.2 lbs = lkg), except for residents with renal or cardiac distress. An excess of fluids can be detrimental for these residents.

5. Survey Procedures

The surveyors are instructed to examine clinical records to determine if residents are being provided with sufficient fluids and are hydrated.

- *Do sampled residents show clinical signs of possible insufficient fluid intake (e.g., dry skin and mucous membranes, cracked lips, poor skin turgor, thirst, fever), abnormal laboratory values (e.g., elevated hemoglobin and hematocrit, potassium, chloride, sodium, albumin, transferrin, blood urea nitrogen (BUN) or urine specific gravity)?*

- *Has the facility provided residents with adequate fluid intake to maintain proper hydration and health?*
    - *If not: Did the facility identify any factors that put the resident at risk of dehydration?*

- *What care did the facility provide to reduce those risk factors and ensure adequate fluid intake (e.g., keep fluids next to the resident at all times and assisting or cuing the resident to drink)? Is staff aware of need for maintaining adequate fluid intake?*

- *If adequate fluid intake is difficult to maintain, have alternative treatment approaches been developed (e.g., attempt to increase fluid intake by the use of popsicles, gelatin, and other similar non-liquid foods)?*

- *Did the MDS trigger RAPs on hydration? What action was taken based on the RAP?*

6. Documentation Guidelines for Hydration

IDT Input: Nursing, dietary

Orders:
Intake and Output
Diagnostic laboratory tests
Fluid restrictions

Care Plan:
Interventions to promote hydration, amount and method of offering fluids, frequency
Nutritional or vitamin supplements
Observation for signs and symptoms of dehydration, episodes of diarrhea or vomiting
Monitoring of intake and output
Contraindications for increased fluid intake due to cardiovascular or renal disease
Target body weight

Progress Notes:

How much and how often fluids are taken, resident cooperation of refusal
Adequacy of fluid intake
Adequacy and tolerance of nutritional intake

Observations of clinical signs and symptom of malnutrition/dehydration:

- pale skin, dull eyes
- red, swollen lips, swollen and/or dry tongue with scarlet or magenta hue
- poor skin turgor, bilateral edema, muscle wasting, calf tenderness
- cachexia
- or reduced ability to take fluids and amount usually consumed

PSYCHOTROPIC DRUGS

Residents in nursing homes have a right to be free from unnecessary drugs. Documentation must include the clinical justification for drug use. For residents suffering from mental illnesses, such as, schizophrenia or depression, the use of psychopharmacological drugs can be both therapeutic and enabling.

Behavioral symptoms should not be **"covered up"** with sedating drugs. First, there should be a systematic assessment to recognize and treat underlying causes of problem behavior. An excellent differential diagnostic process for behavioral symptoms is described in the MDS RAP on Behavioral Symptoms. Social workers should contribute to interdisciplinary care plans by evaluating behaviors to identify underlying causes and by developing alternate non-drug approaches for managing behavior.

1. Federal Regulations

Section 483.25(l) addresses the use of medications, including psychotropic medications.

(l) ***Unnecessary drugs***

(1) General. Each resident's drug regimen must be free from unnecessary drugs. An unnecessary drug is any drug when used:

(i) In excessive dose (including duplicate therapy); or

(ii) For excessive duration; or

(iii) Without adequate monitoring; or

(iv) Without adequate indications for its use; or

(v) In the presence of adverse consequences which indicate the dose should be reduce or discontinued; or

(vi) Any combinations of the reasons above.

(2) Antipsychotic Drugs. Based on a comprehensive assessment of a resident, the facility must ensure that-

(i) Residents who have not used antipsychotic drugs are not given these drugs unless antipsychotic drug therapy is necessary to treat a specific condition as diagnosed and documented in the clinical record; and

(ii) Residents who use antipsychotic drugs receive gradual dose reductions, and behavioral interventions, unless clinically contraindicated, in an effort to discontinue these drugs.

The goal of these regulations and guidelines is to stimulate appropriate differential diagnosis of **"behavioral symptoms"** so the underlying cause of the symptoms is recognized and treated appropriately.

In addition, another goal of these regulations is to prevent the use of psychopharmacological drugs when the **"behavioral symptoms"** is caused by conditions such as:

(1) environmental stressors (e.g., excessive heat, noise, overcrowding, etc)

(2) psychosocial stressors (e.g., abuse, taunting, not allowing a resident's customary daily routine)

(3) treatable medical conditions (e.g., heart disease, diabetes, chronic obstructive pulmonary disease)

2. Quality Measures/Indicators

The following quality measures/indicators are calculated from data submitted on the MDS. Surveyors will review these measures before visiting the facility to identify focus areas for review.

3.1 Use of 9 or more different medications

10.1 Prevalence of antipsychotic use, in the absence of psychotic or related conditions.
10.1-HI High risk
10.1-LO Low risk

10.2 Prevalence of antianxiety/hypnotic use

10.3 Prevalence of hypnotic use more than two times in last week

3. Definitions

The surveyor guidance provides the following definitions:

Unnecessary Drug *A drug used:*

- *in excessive dose (including duplicate drug therapy),*
- *for excessive duration,*

- *without adequate monitoring,*
- *without adequate indicates for use,*
- *in the presence of adverse consequences which indicate the dose should be reduced or discontinued.*

Duplicate Drug Therapy *any drug therapy that duplicates a particular drug effect on the resident. For example, any two or more drugs, whether from the same drug category or not, which have a sedative effect. Duplicate drug therapy should prompt the facility to evaluate the resident for accumulation of the adverse effects.*

Behavioral interventions *modification of the resident's behavior or the resident's environment, including staff approaches to care, to the largest degree possible to accommodate the resident's behavioral symptoms.*

4. Surveyor Guidance

The guidelines to surveyors identify the following categories of drugs for review:

Long acting Benzodiazepines
Benzodiazepines or Other Anxiolytic/Sedative Drugs
Drugs for Sleep Induction
Misc. Hypnotic/Sedative/Anxiolytic Drugs
Antipsychotic Drugs
Antidepressant Drugs

The clinical pharmacist will assist staff with identifying criteria for use, dosages, limitations on duration of use and the need for gradual dose reduction. Documentation is the clinical record must support the clinical indications for the use of the drug.

"Behavioral monitoring charts" are promoted for antipsychotic and benzodiazepine and other anxiolytic/ sedative drugs, but not for antidepressants. This documentation is necessary to assist in:

(1) assessing whether the resident's behavioral symptom is in need of some form of intervention;

(2) determining whether the behavioral symptom is transitory or permanent;

(3) relating the behavioral symptom to other events in the resident's life in order to learn about potential causes (e.g., death in the family, not adhering to the resident's customary daily routine);

(4) ruling out environmental causes such as excessive heat, noise, overcrowding;

(5) ruling out medical causes such as pain, constipation, fever, infection.

For a more complete description of behavioral monitoring charts and how they can assist in the differential diagnosis of behavioral symptoms see the RAP on behavior symptoms.

Diminished sleep in the elderly is not necessarily pathological. Drugs used for sleep induction should only be used if:

- Evidence exists that other possible reasons for insomnia (e.g., depression, pain, noise, light, caffeine) have been ruled out.
- The use of a drug to induce sleep results in the maintenance or improvement of the resident's functional status.

Anxiolytic/Sedative drugs used for purposes other than

sleep induction should have documentation of one of the following indicators:

-- Generalized anxiety disorder
-- Organic mental syndromes (including dementia) with associated agitated states which are quantitatively and objectively documented and which constitute sources of distress or dysfunction to the resident or represent a danger to the resident or others
-- Panic disorders
-- Symptomatic anxiety that occurs in residents with another diagnosed psychiatric disorder (e.g., depression, adjustment disorder)

Antipsychotic drugs should not be used unless the clinical record documents that the resident has one or more of the following "specific conditions."

-- Schizophrenia
-- Schizo-affective disorder
-- Delusional disorder
-- Psychotic mood disorders (including mania and depression with psychotic features)
-- Acute psychotic episodes
-- Brief reactive psychosis
-- Schizophreniform disorder
-- Atypical psychosis
-- Tourette's disorder
-- Huntington's disease

Antipsychotic drugs may be used for organic mental syndromes (now called delirium, dementia, and amnestic and other cognitive disorders by DSM-IV) with associated psychotic and/or agitated behaviors:

a. Which have been quantitatively and objectively

documented (for example, the use of "behavioral monitoring charts")

b. Which are persistent, and

c. Which are not caused by preventable reasons; and

d. Which are causing the resident to:

(1) Present a danger to himself/herself or to others, or

(2) Continuously scream, yell, or pace if these specific behaviors cause an impairment in functional capacity, or

(3) Experience psychotic symptoms (hallucinations, paranoia, delusions) not exhibited as dangerous behaviors or as screaming, yelling, or pacing but which cause the resident distress or impairment in functional capacity.

Antipsychotics should not be used if one or more of the following is/are the <u>only</u> indication:

Wandering;
Poor self care;
Restlessness;
Impaired memory;
Anxiety;
Depression (without psychotic features);
Insomnia;
Unsociability;
Indifference to surroundings;
Fidgeting;
Nervousness;
Uncooperativeness; or
Agitated behaviors that do not represent danger to the resident or others.

For residents using antipsychotic drugs, surveyors are instructed that gradual dose reductions and behavioral interventions may be **"clinically contraindicated"**. A resident <u>need</u>

not undergo a **"gradual dose reduction"** or **"behavioral interventions"** if:

1. The resident has a "specific (psychiatric) condition" and has a history of recurrence of psychotic symptoms (e.g., delusions, hallucinations), which have been stabilized with a maintenance dose of an antipsychotic drug without incurring significant side effects;

2. The resident has organic mental syndrome (now called "Delirium, Dementia, and Amnestic and other Cognitive Disorders" by DSM IV) and has had a gradual dose reduction attempted TWICE in one year and that attempt resulted in the return of symptoms for which the drug was prescribed to a degree that a cessation in the gradual dose reduction, or a return to previous dose reduction was necessary; or

3. The resident's physician provides a justification why the continued use of the drug and the dose of the drug is clinically appropriate. This justification should include:
   (a) a diagnosis, but not simply a diagnostic label or code, but the description of symptoms,
   (b) a discussion of the differential psychiatric and medical diagnosis (e.g., why the resident's behavioral symptom is thought to be a result of a dementia with associated psychosis and/or agitated behaviors, and not the result of an unrecognized painful medical condition of a psychosocial or environmental stressor),
   (c) a description of the justification for the choice of a particular treatment, or treatments, and
   (d) a discussion of why the present dose is necessary to manage the symptoms of the resident. This information need not necessarily be in the physician's progress notes, but must be a part of the resident's clinical record.

The facility assures that residents who are undergoing antipsychotic drug therapy receive adequate monitoring for significant side effects of such therapy with emphasis on the following:

Tardive dyskinesia
Postural (orthostatic) hypotension
Cognitive/behavior impairment
Akathisia
Parkinsonism

The facility is encouraged to initiate therapy with lower doses and when necessary only gradually increase doses. The facility may exceed recommended dosages if it provides evidence to show why it was necessary for the maintenance or improvement in the resident's functional status.

Examples of evidence that would support a justification of why a drug is being used outside these guidelines but in the best interests of the resident may include, but are not limited to:

- A physician's note indicating for example, that the dosage, duration, indication, and monitoring are clinically appropriate, and the reasons why they are clinically appropriate; this note should demonstrate that the physician has care-fully considered the risk/benefit to the resident in using drugs outside the guidelines.

- A medical or psychiatric consultation or evaluation (e.g., Geriatric Depression Scale) that confirms the physician's judgment that use of a drug outside the guidelines is in the best interest of the resident.

- Physician, nursing, or other health professional documentation indicating that the resident is being monitored for adverse consequences or complications of the drug therapy.

- Documentation confirming that previous attempts at dosage reduction have been unsuccessful.

- Documentation (including MDS documentation) showing resident's subjective or objective improvement, or maintenance of function while taking the medication.

- Documentation showing that a resident's decline or deterioration is evaluated by the interdisciplinary team to determine whether a particular drug, or a particular dose, or duration of therapy, may be the cause.

- Documentation showing why the resident's age, weight, or other factors would require a unique drug dose or duration, indication, monitoring.

The facility can refer to a prescriber's (or appropriately trained health professional's) justification as a valid justification for the use of a drug. It may not justify the use of a drug, its dose, its duration, solely on the basis that *"it was ordered"* without supportive information.

5. Survey Procedures for Psychotropic Drugs

The surveyors are to review clinical records of residents using psychotropic drugs to assure appropriate use.

- *Evidence exists that other possible reasons for the resident's distress have been considered and ruled out.*

- *Use results in a maintenance or improvement in the resident's functional status.*

The surveyors are to review clinical records of residents using drugs for sleep induction. Diminished sleep in the elderly is not necessarily pathological. Drugs used for sleep induction should only be used if:

- *Evidence exists that other possible reasons for insomnia (e.g., depression, pain, noise, light, caffeine) have been ruled out and results in maintenance or improvement of resident's functional status.*

6. Documentation Guidelines for Psychotropic Drugs

IDT Input: Nursing, social service, psychologist, psychiatrist, physician

Assessment: Diagnosis justifying use.

Orders: Indicate the specific reason for the use of psychotropic drugs, and a specific time period for use

Care Plan: Goals should focus on maintenance or improvement of behavior
Identify the specific behavior manifestation to be treated.
Steps to rule out possible reasons for resident distress
Alternate behavior management approaches to be used before giving medication
Behavior data to be collected for evaluating effectiveness
Adverse effects to be monitored.
Schedule for dose reductions.

Progress Notes:

Monitoring of specific behavior occurrences, number of times (flow sheets may be used for this)

Describe behavior in objective and observable terms

Evaluate and assess the use of the psychoactive drugs.

- Describe behavior exhibited or behavior controlled
- Possible reasons or circumstances influencing behavior
- Interventions used other than giving the medication
- Resident response and tolerance

Data regarding behavior manifestation, frequency and type
Observations for adverse effects

RESTRAINTS

Residents in nursing facilities have a right to be free from physical restraints that do not assist the resident to attain a higher level of functioning. Medical symptoms that warrant the use of restraints should be reflected in comprehensive assessment and care planning. It is further expected that the facility engage in a systematic and gradual process toward reducing restraints. For those residents whose care plans indicate the need for restraints, gradually increasing the time for ambulation or muscle strengthening activities could be considered.

For the resident or family to make an informed choice about the use of restraints, the facility should explain to the resident the negative outcomes of restraint use. Potential negative outcomes include incontinence, decreased range of motion, decreased ability to ambulate, symptoms of withdrawal or depression, and reduced social contact. However, the surrogate or representative cannot give permission to use restraints for the sake of discipline or staff convenience or when the restraint is not necessary to treat the residents medical symptoms.

1. Federal Regulations

Section 483.13(a) addresses the use of physical restraints.

The resident has the right to be free from any physical or chemical restraints imposed for purposes of discipline or convenience, and not required to treat the resident's medical symptoms.

The intent of this requirement is for each person to attain and maintain his/her highest practicable well-being in an environment that prohibits the use of restraints for discipline or convenience and limits restraint use to circumstances in which the resident has medical symptoms that warrant the use of restraints.

2. Quality Measures/Indicators

The following quality measures/indicators are calculated from data submitted on the MDS. Surveyors will review these indicators before visiting the facility to identify focus areas for review.

11.1 Residents who are physically restrained

3. Definitions

The guidance to surveyors provide the following definitions.

Physical Restraints

Any manual method or physical or mechanical device, material, or equipment attached or adjacent to the resident's body that the individual cannot remove easily which restricts freedom of movement or normal access to one's body.

Physical restraints include, but are not limited to, leg restraints, arm restraints, hand mitts, soft ties or vests, lap cushions, and lap trays the resident cannot remove easily. Also included as restraints are facility practices that meet the definition of a restraint, such as:

- Using side rails that keep a resident from voluntarily getting out of bed;
- Tucking in or using velcro to hold a sheet, fabric, or clothing tightly so that a resident's movement is

restricted;

- Using devices in conjunction with a chair, such as trays, tables, bars or belts, that the resident cannot remove easily, that prevent the resident from rising;
- Placing a resident in a chair that prevents a resident from rising; and
- Placing a chair or bed so close to a wall that the wall prevents the resident from rising out of the chair or voluntarily getting out of bed.

Side rails sometimes restrain residents. The use of side rails as restraints is prohibited unless they are necessary to treat a resident's medical symptoms. Residents who attempt to exit a bed through, between, over or around side rails are at risk of injury or death. The potential for serious injury is more likely from a fall from a bed with raised side rails than from a fall from a bed where side rails are not used. They also potentially increase the likelihood that the resident will spend more time in bed and fall when attempting to transfer from the bed. As with other restraints, for residents who are restrained by side rails, it is expected that the process facilities employ to reduce the use of side rails as restraints is systematic and gradual to ensure the resident's safety while treating the resident's medical symptom.

The same device may have the effect of restraining one individual but not another, depending on the individual resident's condition and circumstances. For example, partial rails may assist one resident to enter and exit the bed independently while acting as a restraint for another.

An enclosed framed wheeled walker, with or without a posterior seat, would not meet the definition of a restraint if the resident could easily open the front gate and exit the device. If the resident cannot open the front gate (due to cognitive or physical limitations that prevent him or her from exiting the device or because the device has been altered to prevent the resident from exiting the device), the enclosed framed wheeled walker would meet the definition of a restraint since the device would restrict the resident's freedom of movement (e.g. transferring to another chair, to the commode, or into the bed). The decision on whether framed wheeled walkers are a restraint must be made on an individual basis.

4. Surveyor Guidance

The facility should explain to the resident or responsible person how the use of restraints would treat the resident's medical symptoms and assist the resident in attaining or maintaining his/her highest practicable level of physical or psychological well-being. In addition, the facility must also explain the potential negative outcomes of restraint use which include, but are not limited to, declines in the resident's physical functioning (e.g., ability to ambulate) and muscle condition, contractures, increased incidence of infections and development of pressure sores/ulcers, delirium, agitation, and incontinence.

Moreover, restraint use may constitute an accident hazard. Restraints have been found in some cases to increase the incidence of falls or head trauma due to falls and other accidents (e.g., strangulation, entrapment).

Finally, residents who are restrained may face a loss of autonomy, dignity and self respect, and may show symptoms of withdrawal, depression, or reduced social contact. In effect, restraint use can reduce independence, functional capacity, and quality of life. Alternatives to restraint use should be considered and discussed with the resident.

5. Survey Procedures

Surveyors will examine clinical records to determine if the use of restraints is for the therapeutic benefit of the resident and if the facility follows a systematic process of evaluation and care planning prior to using restraints.

- *What are the medical symptoms that led to the consideration of the use of restraints?*

- *Are these symptoms caused by failure to:*
  - -- *Meet individual needs in accordance with MDS Section AC, Customary Daily Routines*
  - -- *Use rehabilitative/restorative care?*
  - -- *Provide meaningful activities?*
  - -- *Manipulate the resident's environment, including seating?*

- *Can the cause(s) of the medical symptoms be eliminated or reduced?*

- *If the cause(s) cannot be eliminated or reduced, then has the facility attempted to use alternatives in order to avoid a decline in physical functioning associated with restraint use?*

- *If alternatives have been tried and deemed unsuccessful, does the facility use the least restrictive restraint for the least amount of time? Does the facility monitor and adjust care to reduce the potential for negative outcomes while continually trying to find and use less restrictive alternatives?*

- *Did the resident or legal surrogate make an informed choice about the use of restraints? Were risks, benefits, and alternatives explained?*

- *Does the facility use the Physical Restraints RAP to evaluate the appropriateness of restraint use?*

- *Has the facility re-evaluated the need for the restraint, made efforts to eliminate its use and maintained residents' strength and mobility?*

Use of side rails should be assessed in the clinical record whether or not they are being used as a restraint. When used for mobility or transfer, assessment should include a review of the resident's:

- *Bed mobility (e.g., would the use of a device assist the resident to turn from side to side? Is the resident totally immobile and unable to change position without assistance?); and*

- *Ability to transfer between positions, to and from bed or chair, to stand and toilet (e.g., does the raised side rail add risk to the resident's ability to transfer?).*

6. Documentation Guidelines for Physical Restraints

IDT Input: Nursing, activity, social services, physical therapy, occupational therapy

Orders: Specific reason (medical symptom) for the use of physical restraints
Type of restraint
When to apply

Assessment: Medical symptom that requires use
Frequent of use, how long resident is in restraints, time of day use
Response of resident to restraints
Potential risks and benefits of restraint use
Options and alternatives to restraint use, such as, modifying the resident's environment and/or routine.

Care Plan: Medical symptom for which restraints are used
Method of application, specific period to be used, part of the body to be supported

Schedule for turning and repositioning, provision for exercise periods free of restraint
Restorative care to enhance abilities to stand, transfer, and walk safely
Devices, such as a trapeze, to increase a resident's mobility in bed
Placing the bed lower to the floor and surrounding the bed with a soft mat
Alarms that monitor attempts to arise
Frequent monitoring by staff with periodic assisted toileting for residents who attempt to arise to use the bathroom
Visual and verbal reminders to use the call bell
Alternate approaches to be used before restraints applied
A process to reduce the use of restraints that is systematic and gradual to ensure the resident's safety while treating the resident's medical symptom
Meaningful activity programs and pursuits
Family, volunteer and one to one interventions

Progress Notes:

Flow sheet documentation of application of physical restraints
Release and repositioning
Informed choice given by resident or responsible person
Reports to activity programs and pursuits
Frequency and response to visits from family, volunteers, one to one.
Evaluation for risks, decline in functioning, pressure ulcers, incontinence, withdrawal

References

CMS Online Manual System, Skilled Nursing Facilities, Pub 100-07, State Operations Manual, Rev 12 10-14-05, www.cms.hhs.gov/manuals.

RAI User's Manual, MDS 2.0, Rev. December 2005, and Quality Measures, www.cms.hhs.gov/nursinghomequalityinits.
